The UK Association of Supportive Care in Cancer Handbook of Supportive Oncology

What does supportive oncology do that palliative care doesn't already do? Answering that question forms part of the rationale behind this text. Supportive oncology is delivered across the whole cancer experience from diagnosis through treatment to post-treatment care, and so necessitates the involvement of most clinical specialties and many non-clinical services. Palliative care – which focuses on advanced disease and end of life – has a special and important role within this broader and longer-term scope of supportive care in cancer.

This handbook defines the new and emerging specialty of supportive oncology and equips the workforce with the appropriate skill sets:

- Providing personalized and targeted treatments consistent with the stage of disease
- A focus on preservation and improvement in quality of life
- Affecting survival and the quality of that survival
- Permitting the use of the most effective anti-cancer agents
- Assisting in accurate diagnosis and management

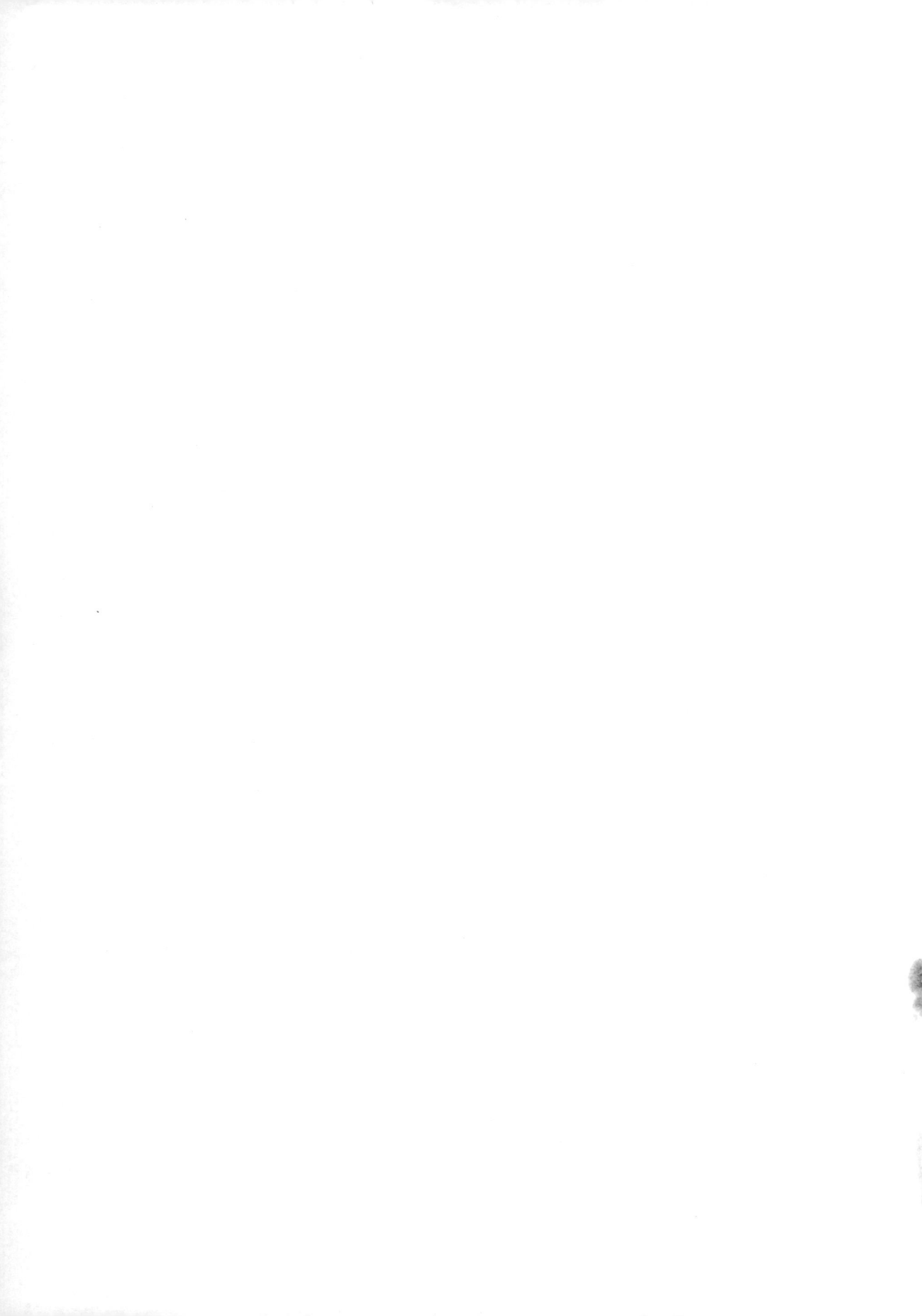

The UK Association of Supportive Care in Cancer Handbook of Supportive Oncology

Edited by

Richard Berman FRCP

Consultant in Supportive & Palliative Care,
The Christie NHS Foundation Trust
Honorary Senior Lecturer in Cancer Sciences,
University of Manchester, UK

Ben Heyworth BA

Survivorship Network Manager,
The Christie NHS Foundation Trust
Honorary Lecturer, University of Manchester, UK

Ashique Ahamed MRCP

Consultant in Supportive & Palliative Care,
The Christie NHS Foundation Trust, Manchester, UK

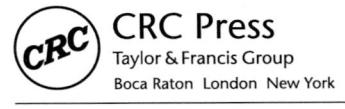

CRC Press
Taylor & Francis Group
Boca Raton London New York

CRC Press is an imprint of the
Taylor & Francis Group, an **informa** business

Designed cover image: Getty Images

First edition published 2025
by CRC Press
2385 NW Executive Center Drive, Suite 320, Boca Raton FL 33431

and by CRC Press
4 Park Square, Milton Park, Abingdon, Oxon, OX14 4RN

CRC Press is an imprint of Taylor & Francis Group, LLC

© 2025 selection and editorial matter, Richard Berman, Ben Heyworth, and Ashique Ahamed; individual chapters, the contributors

ISBN: 9781032440095 (hbk)
ISBN: 9781032440088 (pbk)
ISBN: 9781003369912 (ebk)

DOI: 10.1201/9781003369912

Typeset in Palatino
by Deanta Global Publishing Services, Chennai, India

Contents

Section IV   Special Populations

Section V   Organizational Changes

Contributors

Sam H. Ahmedzai
University of Sheffield
Sheffield, UK

Malcolm Brown
Ulster University
Belfast, Northern Ireland, UK

James Burtonwood
University Hospitals Bristol NHS
   Foundation Trust
Bristol, UK

Joanne Collins
The Christie NHS Foundation Trust
Manchester, UK

Tim Cooksley
The Christie NHS Foundation Trust
Manchester, UK

Tasha Critchlow
Royal Marsden Hospital
London, UK

Emma Dillsworth
Royal Surrey NHS Foundation Trust
Surrey, UK

Lisa Durrant
Beacon Radiotherapy Centre
Taunton, UK

Fabio Gomes
The Christie NHS Foundation Trust
Manchester, UK

Emma Hallam
Nottingham University Hospitals NHS
   Trust
Nottingham, UK

Lesley Howells
Maggie's Lead Psychologist and Consultant
   Clinical Psychologist Maggie's
London, UK

Freya Howle
The Christie NHS Foundation Trust
Manchester, UK

Victoria Jones
Pennine Care NHS Foundation Trust
Ashton under Lyne, UK

Emily Kellett
Countess of Chester NHS Foundation Trust
Chester, UK

Charlotte Leach
Royal Surrey NHS Foundation Trust
Surrey, UK

Laura Miller
Nottingham University Hospitals NHS
   Trust
Nottingham, UK

Oli Minton
University Hospitals Sussex NHS
   Foundation Trust
Sussex, UK

Dan Monnery
Clatterbridge Cancer Centre NHS
   Foundation Trust
Liverpool, UK

Simon Noble
Cardiff University
Cardiff, UK

Anna Olsson-Brown
University Hospitals Sussex NHS
    Foundation Trust
Sussex, UK

Bob Philips
Hull York Medical School
Heslington, UK

Martine Puts
University of Toronto
Toronto, Canada

Hanna Simpson
The Christie NHS Foundation Trust
Manchester, UK

Jo Thompson
Royal Surrey NHS Foundation Trust
Surrey, UK

Jennifer Vidrine
Newcastle upon Tyne Hospitals NHS
    Foundation Trust
Newcastle upon Tyne, UK

Section I

Setting the Scene

1

Introduction

Richard Berman, Emily Kellett, and Sam H. Ahmedzai

What Is Supportive Oncology and Where Did It Come from?

> Supportive care is provided to people with cancer and their carers throughout the patient pathway, from pre-diagnosis onwards. It should be given equal priority with other aspects of care and be fully integrated with diagnosis and treatment.[1]

Twenty years ago, the NHS first presented oncologists with the challenge of integrating supportive care into the emerging clinical and organizational pathways in oncology. This was through the 2004 publication of the NICE guideline *Improving Supportive and Palliative Care for Adults with Cancer.*

This far-seeing document introduced the phrase 'supportive care' in oncology and cited the definition from the National Council for Hospice and Specialist Palliative Care Services (NCHSPCS): It is care

> that helps the patient and their family to cope with cancer and treatment of it – from pre-diagnosis, through the process of diagnosis and treatment, to cure, continuing illness or death and into bereavement. It helps the patient to maximise the benefits of treatment and to live as well as possible with the effects of the disease. It is given equal priority alongside diagnosis and treatment.

This definition was, in fact, appropriated from the Multinational Association for the Supportive Care in Cancer (MASCC), an already established and extremely influential voice.[2] Founded in 1990, MASCC remains the largest global supportive care organization, and now includes members in over 70 countries around the world. In 1998 MASCC joined forces with the International Society of Oral Oncology (ISOO), an organization that addresses the management of complications arising in oral tissues secondary to cancer and its treatments. MASCC and ISOO hold a joint Annual Meeting each June where the latest ideas and research in supportive care are showcased.

The publication of the NICE 2004 guidance raised a burning question amongst oncologists as well as existing providers of palliative care (including the specialty of palliative medicine), and NHS structures providing cancer services – "What does supportive care do that palliative care doesn't already do?" That question has been hotly debated for two decades and indeed forms one of the rationales for this handbook.

DOI: 10.1201/9781003369912-2

The answer to this question was already evident in the NICE guidance itself, which recommended that supportive care should encompass a wide range of diverse disciplines and practices, ranging from symptom management, to rehabilitation, to social, spiritual, and psychological support, patient information, and complementary therapies.

Supportive care is, therefore, delivered across the whole cancer experience from diagnosis through treatment to post-treatment care, and so necessitates the involvement of most clinical specialties and many non-clinical services.

Palliative care – which focuses on advanced disease and end of life – has a special place within the broader and longer-term scope of supportive care in cancer. However, innovative practitioners increasingly recognize that palliative care services alone – as they are applied in most parts of the world – can no longer deliver on the additional multiple challenges of providing care to people across the entire spectrum of the disease, or for the growing number of cancer survivors.

Palliative care has an important and well-established role in the advanced stages of cancer. There are examples of palliative care teams which have embraced supportive care in cancer and other long-term conditions, but this is not currently the norm in many Western countries. Furthermore, the skill set for the management of advanced disease and end of life does not meet the challenges of those who may now live for many years with incurable but treatable disease, those with acute post-surgical pain, or the multifaceted toxicities of chemotherapy, immunotherapy, targeted therapies, or endocrine and radiation therapies. Section II, Chapter 2 discusses the emergence of a recent subspecialization of cancer care – acute oncology – in which supportive care works alongside oncologists to take on these challenges of early complications and toxicities.

It is important to state clearly that supportive oncology is not an alternative or competitor to palliative care. Indeed, up till now the large majority of those practicing clinical supportive care have come from 'traditional' palliative care backgrounds. Most of these – from all disciplines – still have a 'day job' delivering conventional evidence-based palliative care for patients with advancing disease and at the end of life.

But the reason for this handbook is that we are now living in a world where cancer treatments are rapidly advancing, where many more people are living longer with or beyond the disease. This means that we must be poised to recognize a new and emerging speciality, one which provides care consistent with the stages of disease and delivered through the entire cancer continuum. This speciality needs a new workforce with appropriate skill sets. Supportive oncology clinicians must have the broad range of skills needed to provide day-to-day care across the whole spectrum of the disease, with critical elements from the main associated allied non-oncology specialties. Professor Richard Gralla, a US-based pioneer in supportive oncology, suggests that the clinical care must aim to:

- Provide personalized and targeted treatments consistent with the stage of disease
- Focus on preservation and improvement in quality of life
- Affect survival and the quality of that survival
- Permit the use of the most effective anti-cancer agents
- Assist accurate diagnosis and management

Why Are We Using the Term 'Supportive Oncology'?

Semantics have played an import role in the evolution of supportive and palliative care. In the early days of the modern hospice movement in the 1960s–1970s, the term evolved from 'terminal care' to 'hospice care' and only in the 1980s did 'palliative care' seriously enter the vocabulary. Even near the millennium, many from traditional hospice services argued against 'palliative care' as it took away the focus on the last period of life and because it threatened to 'medicalize' death and dying.[3] Now of course, the terms palliative care and palliative medicine are universally accepted for services for advanced stages of disease.

After the 2004 NICE guideline for 'supportive care' in cancer, a new debate emerged with some palliative care providers objecting to the notion that their role was limited to only 2 of 13 recommendations. But they had initially failed to appreciate that the new supportive care agenda was much wider than the advanced stages of cancer.

This handbook argues for another seismic semantic change – to accept the key role that supportive care now has in the delivery of both 'high tech' and compassionate care for people going through all the stages of cancer. Just as oncology itself has broken down to subspecialties covering diagnostics, surgery, drug-based treatments, and radiation-based treatments, this handbook argues that we should recognize the emerging contribution of supportive care alongside those workforces. This is 'supportive oncology'.

As well as providing the original definition of supportive care, MASCC also adopted the strapline "supportive care makes excellent cancer care possible". We endorse that and believe that recognizing supportive oncology in the UK as an aspiring new division of oncology will increase its recognition in the wider healthcare communities, including policy and funding.

The UK Association of Supportive Care in Cancer (UKASCC) defines supportive oncology as (adapted from the MASCC definition):

> The coordinated contributions of a collective group of medical and non-medical specialties that collectively help to prevent and manage the adverse effects of cancer and its treatment. Supportive oncology spans the entire spectrum of the disease. It includes prehabilitation, management of treatable but incurable cancer, curable disease, cancer survivorship and palliative and end of life care.

The Changing Populations of Cancer

The diagnostic and therapeutic capabilities of cancer care are rapidly evolving, and as a result new populations of cancer patients are discernible. Increasingly, oncological advances are reported as success stories of modern medicine and have resulted in an increasing number of people, at different stages of their illness, who are living with and beyond their initial cancer prognosis. Indeed, for many people cancer has become a long-term condition. The number of people now living with cancer is having a significant impact on the nature and volume of health and social care required.

For many people, cancer treatment is very successful, and they tolerate treatments well. However, at least 25% of people living with cancer and those living after cancer treatment in the UK will have one or more physical or psychosocial consequences affecting their lives on a long-term basis.[4] The result is a greater demand for rehabilitation and support services needed to manage the long-term effects of cancer and its treatment.

The UK charity Macmillan Cancer Support estimates that there are currently 3 million people living with cancer in the UK, and this is set to rise to 4 million by 2030 and to 5.3 million by 2040.[5] Over the past ten years, rates of cancer mortality have decreased on average across the UK; around half of those diagnosed with cancer today will live for at least ten years after their diagnosis. More than one in three people who have had cancer (35%) will now ultimately die from another cause.[4] 'Living with and beyond cancer' (LWBC) is a term that has been used for many years to describe this population. The issues facing LWBC survivors and those with late consequences of earlier cancer treatments, respectively, are discussed in Section III (Chapter 5).

Because of the increase in treatment options for patients who have relapsed after earlier responses to anti-cancer treatments, a new category is being recognized: Those who have 'treatable but not curable cancer'. Several types of cancer now fall into this category, including CLL, CML, multiple myeloma, pleural mesothelioma, and several types of secondary cancers including breast, brain, and lung.

A retrospective study in 2021 by White et al. estimated that 110,615 people in England are living with managed but incurable disease with an additional 51,946 in their last year of life and a further 57,117 people identified as at high risk of cancer recurrence.[6] Many of these patients will have a significantly longer prognosis, perhaps years, than previously, or it has been proposed that they be considered as a new class of 'metastatic cancer survivors'.[7]

Although metastatic disease has conventionally fallen into the domain of palliative care, to address the needs of those with managed but incurable disease, who are still attending hospital for novel treatment options, would pose a significant challenge for the traditional palliative care approach, which largely focuses on care within the last 12 months of life.

Populations Served by Supportive Oncology

The new concept of supportive oncology encompasses all people with cancer, at any stage of the disease. Supportive oncology starts at the point of diagnosis, continues through treatment, extends into remission, and encompasses those people at the end of life. Like other areas of medicine, a personalized care model, which is focused on the needs of patients and ideally of their families, is essential.

This patient population is, therefore, evolving as advances in oncology continue to extend life. Some of the same clinicians who provide end of life care are also – in specific settings – broadening the scope of their work to include other parts of the cancer continuum, including cancer survivorship. See Section V (Chapter 8) for more on the overlap between supportive and palliative care in advanced disease.

People undergoing cancer treatment will have different needs and priorities compared to people who are in remission or those nearing the end of life. There will inevitably be variation in physical, emotional, psychological, and social concerns, and treatment may switch between active cancer treatment, remission, relapse, and back again.

Furthermore, with the advent of newer treatments, supportive oncology will continue to change and adapt into the future. Novel therapies bring novel side effects, and optimal supportive oncology requires input from multiple medical specialties, and allied health services, to assist accurate diagnosis and management of these, and ultimately improve outcomes.

Prehabilitation before surgery or other therapies is a supportive oncology development that is relatively new but is already being incorporated into treatment pathways. Physiotherapy and occupational therapy are essential components of this and post-treatment rehabilitation. Patient optimization and rehabilitation are discussed in Section III (Chapter 5).

Measuring Patient Needs and Outcomes

Given the large and growing populations of patients who could benefit from supportive oncology and with the current limited workforce and resources, the important question is – how do we measure who should receive supportive care and how do we assess the impact of services?

One key but overlooked part of the NICE 2004 guidance in 'Improving supportive and palliative care for adults with cancer' was in the section on 'general palliative care services'. This referred to the important provision for 'accurate holistic assessment of patient needs'. Holistic needs assessment (HNA) is indeed not only relevant for patients with advanced disease and at the end of life, but also for patients at the start of cancer treatment, after its completion, and at key stages afterwards, including at the transition to palliative and end of life care.

Oncology services have been at the forefront globally in embracing the use of patient-reported outcome measures (PROMs) to evaluate people's experiences in relation to their health, their disease, and their healthcare journey.[8] Measuring quality of life outcomes after cancer treatment is now embedded in most clinical trials from Phase 2 onwards, and it should also be incorporated into supportive oncology evaluation. Numerous cancer-specific tools are available such as the EORTC QLQ-C30, which has multiple modules for assessing outcomes in different types of cancer, or after different treatment modalities.[9] More generic instruments such as Euroqol EQ-5D contain less detail on cancer-specific outcomes but have the advantage of yielding data that are comparable with other diseases.

NHS England and NHS Digital have now adopted a national cancer quality of life dashboard, which also uses EQ-5D. It is important that such metrics are in future applied to all patients to demonstrate the role of supportive oncology in maintaining and optimizing their quality of life. Additionally, the use of cancer-specific tools is important to identify patient priorities at specific points in time and help identify the range of pertinent biopsychosocial issues. Thus, they may be effective in helping to direct the most impactful interventions of a supportive oncology service.

How Long Does Supportive Oncology Intervention Last?

The length of time that a supportive oncology service could impact on a patient's illness trajectory will be variable. Many people will become symptom- or even cancer-free but still encounter late-onset consequences of treatment which could adversely affect their ultimate recovery. Others will require increasing input from supportive oncology services as their disease progresses.

Comprehensive supportive oncology will require a patient-directed and flexible approach, changing dynamically according to the changing severity of illness and clinical need. This will apply to assessment of needs and outcomes, as well as for management that is consistent with stage of disease.

Critically, how patients are assessed and referred to a supportive oncology service, subsequently discharged, and possibly re-referred later on will also depend on the structure and capacity of that service, what is offered, and how it can address the needs of the patients. Such a service would need to be adaptive, multidisciplinary, and responsive to the broad range of needs of a growing and increasingly diverse patient group. These factors are especially relevant as supportive oncology moves into teenage and young adult (TYA) populations, geriatric populations, and other diverse groups. Section IV discusses these special groups.

Service Models and Workforce Requirements for Supportive Oncology

A range of different service models have been developed which encompass some of the fundamental aspects of supportive oncology. These include acute oncology, integrative oncology, enhanced supportive care, geriatric oncology, and survivorship clinics.[9] The delivery of these services that provide what may be considered under the umbrella of "supportive oncology" varies across organizations and institutions, with wide variety in terms of target population, access mechanisms, leadership, and staff involved. Until there is a future national policy on supportive oncology, it is likely these services will develop idiosyncratically and be largely based within larger cancer centres, dependant on the expertise and enthusiasm of early adopters.

Although the ideal model is yet to be defined, based on work in palliative and supportive care in cancer,[9] the development and delivery of high-quality supportive oncology services are likely to require several key components delivered by a multidisciplinary and multi-professional team through a holistic and personalized lens.

Timely access to a multidisciplinary team provides patients and their families with individualized specialist involvement. The multidisciplinary team is usually comprised of doctors, nurses, pharmacists, psychological support teams, and allied health professionals including, but not limited to, physiotherapists, occupational therapists, dieticians and nutritionists, speech and language therapists, social workers, financial support teams, chaplains, art therapists, and music therapists. The specialist doctors involved in the multidisciplinary team may include tumour-specific oncology physicians and surgeons, acute oncology teams, general and specialist medical physicians (including endocrinologists, cardiologists, respiratory physicians, etc.), radiologists, and palliative care physicians. Each member contributes to the development of a coordinated care plan, based on the needs of the individual patient. This team approach not only benefits the patient and his/her family but also improves the delivery of care through a reduction in professional burnout and shared responsibility and decision making.[10]

**CASE STUDY 1: CLATTERBRIDGE CANCER CENTRE
– ENHANCED SUPPORTIVE CARE (ESC)**

The Enhanced Supportive Care (ESC) service at the Clatterbridge Cancer Centre began in 2016 as part of the national NHS England Commissioning for Quality and Innovation (CQUIN) to establish ESC services within cancer care in England. The initial aim of the service was to integrate early access to palliative care and other supportive care specialties as early as possible in the care of patients with treatable but not curable cancer. The initial pilot ran three outpatient clinics a week focusing on patients with central nervous system, head and neck, hepatobiliary, and melanoma primary malignancies.

As the service developed, driven by evidence of improved outcomes including improved patient symptom burden, reduced secondary care requirements, cost savings, and positive patient and family experience, expansion to other patient groups included:

- All primary tumour groups in 2020
- Patients receiving curative treatment in 2021
- Patients with late effects of previous treatment in 2022

Currently, the ESC service at CCC delivers 14 outpatient clinics per week across 3 hospital sites. Two clinics are embedded within the primary oncology clinics for hepatobiliary and lung malignancies to enable same-day supportive care access when patients see their oncologist. One clinic is exclusively for late effects. The team also delivers an ambulatory service 11am–7pm Monday to Friday for any patients, including those receiving curative treatment, to access same-day emergency symptom control and support. Patients typically receive an initial holistic assessment from a palliative care practitioner who acts both as a clinician and care navigator, linking the patient in with the required elements of the wider supportive care MDT. The ESC service uses a shared governance structure to combine the oversight and strategic leadership of all supportive care specialties including therapies, nutrition, psycho-oncology, prehabilitation, toxicity management, and palliative care within one clinical group. These teams also have a shared education and research agenda and clinically interface via a weekly MDT to facilitate patient care. More patients each year use the ESC service, with 1,399 patients using this service in 2023–24.

To provide equitable and accessible care for all patients living with a cancer diagnosis, a high-quality supportive oncology service needs systems to define the target patient population, interventions, and outcomes, all of which must be tailored to the local patient population and available resources. Traditionally patients have been referred by oncology teams to services providing aspects of supportive oncology, of which there may be many within single organizations. This approach however can be subjective and result in issues of equity in terms of access.

A proactive approach to supportive oncology involves early identification of patients' needs with easy access to the expert best placed to manage those needs. Underpinning this is a recognition that the identification and management of the adverse effects of cancer and its treatment differ depending on where the patient is along their cancer journey. The management of pain at end of life is very different from the management of pain in patients who are "cured" from cancer. In addition, patients' needs may fluctuate over time, depending on the effects of the cancer itself, the treatment options, and existing comorbidities.[11]

CASE STUDY 2: THE CHRISTIE NHS FOUNDATION TRUST – SUPPORTIVE ONCOLOGY DIRECTORATE

The Christie Directorate of Supportive Oncology is the UK first to recognize all "supportive services" in one place. Launched in 2024, the purpose of the directorate is to fully integrate multidisciplinary supportive oncology within elective and non-elective pathways, and input into outpatient management and follow up.

The supportive oncology directorate aims to:

1) Ensure equity of access for all patients to services that will enhance people's experience and quality of life during and after treatment
2) Increase better access and decrease waits for clinical expertise
3) Increase Senior Medical and Allied Health input into hotline, ward, and outpatient provision
4) Through the above activity, decrease non-elective admissions to hospital and influence a reduction in length of stay overall

The model of care provided by the directorate spans the full requirement of patients (across seven days) via an integrated medical model aligned with acute oncology. This includes attending ward rounds, the provision of hotline advice and guidance, daily drop-in supportive oncology clinics, and shared MDT discussion of complex patients. The approach aims to avoid the need for hospital admission by inputting into 'Front Door' services at the Christie, to help patients when GPs and other secondary care services are not accessible other than through A&E (emergency room).

An ideal conceptual model of supportive oncology would involve a reorganization of systems and processes to inform joined-up cohesive working with the efficient use of clinic space and resources, using wherever appropriate virtual consultations to reduce the number of burdensome clinical attendances for patients and their families. This would require clear real-time communication and information sharing between services, patients and families, and healthcare professionals. Novel approaches to support optimal communication are being tested in clinical practice such as video-consultations,[12] digital urgent care planning systems,[13] and virtual care.[14]

The UK Association of Supportive Care in Cancer (UKASCC)

UKASCC's vision is to "promote excellence in the care of all those directly and indirectly affected by cancer in all four countries of the UK", by inspiring the workforce through the support of professionals in their research, practice and learning and development.

Established as a registered charity in 2021, the organisation provides an annual supportive oncology conference, hosts a new Royal College of Radiology endorsed clinical fellowship programme, and acts to promote supportive oncology nationally, and by supporting research.

References

1. NICE. Improving supportive and palliative care for adults with cancer, *Guideline* [internet], 2004; available at: https://www.nice.org.uk/guidance/csg4.
2. Multinational Association of Supportive Care in Cancer; available at: https://mascc.org/.
3. Clark D et al. *New Themes in Palliative Care*. McGraw-Hill Education; 1977.
4. Macmillan Cancer Support. Cured but at what cost [internet], 2013; available at: www.macmillan.org.uk/dfsmedia/1a6f23537f7f4519bb0cf14c45b2a629/14614-10061/cured-but-at-what-cost-summary-report-july-2013 (accessed Sept 2024).
5. Macmillan Fact Sheet [internet], 2024; available at: www.macmillan.org.uk/dfsmedia/1a6f23537f7f4519bb0cf14c45b2a629/16768-10061/Cancer-statistics-fact-sheet-April-2024 (accessed Sept 2024).
6. White R et al. Treatable but not curable cancer in England: a retrospective cohort study using cancer registry data and linked data sets. *BMJ Open*. 2021;11(1).
7. Lai-Kwon J et al. Evolving landscape of metastatic cancer survivorship: reconsidering clinical care, policy, and research priorities for the modern era. *J Clin Oncol*. 2023;41(18):3304-3310.
8. Di Maio M et al. The role of patient-reported outcome measures in the continuum of cancer clinical care: ESMO clinical practice guideline. 2022. *Ann Oncol*. 2022;33(9):978–892.
9. EORTC, Questionnaire QLQ-C30 [internet], 1993; available at: https://qol.eortc.org/questionnaires/core/eortc-qlq-c30/ (accessed Sept 2024).
10. Hui D et al. Models of supportive care in oncology. *Curr Opin Oncol*. 2021;33(4):259–266.
11. Hui D et al. Improving patient and caregiver outcomes in oncology: team-based, timely, and targeted palliative care. *CA: Cancer J Clinic*. 2018;68(5):356–376.
12. Cascella M et al. Satisfaction with telemedicine for cancer pain management: a model of care and cross-sectional patient satisfaction study. *Curr Oncol*. 2022;29(8):5566–5578.
13. Orlovic M et al. Impact of advance care planning on dying in hospital: evidence from urgent care records. *PLoS One* 2020;15(12).
14. Pham Q et al. Virtual care for prostate cancer survivorship: protocol for an evaluation of a nurse-led algorithm-enhanced virtual clinic implemented at five cancer centres across Canada. *BMJ Open*. 2021;11(4).

Section II

Clinical Challenges for Supportive Oncology

2

Managing Treatment and Cancer-Related Acute Issues – Acute Oncology

Tim Cooksley

Introduction

In the UK patients with cancer account for around 15% of all acute inpatient stays and the delivery of acute care consumes nearly half of the spending on patients with cancer.[1] Cancer care has become increasingly specialized and advances in therapy have resulted in a larger number of patients receiving care as an outpatient. As a result of these advances in care and the increasing number of patients receiving cancer therapies, there has been a significant increase in the number of patients presenting with unscheduled cancer-related emergencies.[2]

The management of acute oncology patients presents many challenges. The increase in immunotherapy and targeted therapy have not only altered prognosis for some cancers but also produce a wide range of toxicity which requires expert management. Early recognition of acutely unwell cancer patients at risk of clinical deterioration is important not only to instigate treatment but also to facilitate decisions regarding whether escalation of care and cardiopulmonary resuscitation is appropriate.[3] This requires an understanding of the patient's underlying prognosis and goals of care, which often requires oncological advice.

In the UK, there have been two strategies adopted to improve the care of acutely unwell cancer patients – the development of specialist admission units in tertiary cancer units and the evolution of "acute oncology services" to support patients admitted to non-cancer hospitals.

Acute Oncology Services

In 2009, following a series of reports recognizing that a significant proportion of cancer patients presenting to UK Emergency Departments (ED) received sub-optimal care, the UK National Chemotherapy Advisory Group (NCAG) recommended that every UK hospital with an emergency department should establish an acute oncology service.[4] As a result of the varying demands and resources available across the UK to develop acute oncology services at each hospital there has been a wide range of models employed to deliver this strategy. The core of all acute oncology teams has been an acute oncology specialist nurse co-ordinating the service often supported by visiting oncologists.

The fundamental principles of an acute oncology service are to promote education, awareness, and early access to specialist oncology input. It aims to drive integrated working between acute care physicians, surgeons, medical specialists, and oncologists. Acute oncology supports the variety of emergency presentations including initial diagnosis, treatment complications, and end-of-life issues. These encompass the three clearly defined types of acute oncology presentation:

Type 1 – patients who present with a new diagnosis of cancer

Type 2 – patients who present with toxicities related to cancer treatments

Type 3 – patients who present symptoms and complications related to the cancer itself

Despite many national initiatives targeting early diagnosis of cancer in the UK, around a quarter of new cancers continue to be diagnosed during an emergency admission.[5] This number has been increased by the COVID-19 pandemic and the recent long waiting times have further exacerbated this problem. These patients are at risk of poorly co-ordinated care with late referrals to oncology and palliative care services. Acute oncology services have played a fundamental role in supporting the management of these patients and ensuring diagnostic pathways are completed in a timely fashion. This is especially pertinent in patients presenting with malignancy of unknown origin (MUO) who often experience fractured diagnostic journeys with a lack of continuity and clinical accountability.[6]

A year review of a regional network acute oncology service covering 7 hospitals in the Northwest of England reported 3013 new patient admissions of which 19% were type 1 admissions, 30% type 2, and 51% type 3.[7] Acute oncology models reduced the length of inpatient hospital stays and delivered significant cost savings.[7,8]

Ambulatory Care

Ambulatory care is recognized as a key tenet in ensuring the safety and sustainability of acute care services. The fundamental basis for ambulatory care is that patients presenting with acute illnesses can be stratified as low risk for developing complications and therefore do not require traditional inpatient care.[9] The NHS targets that 25% of all acute medical presentations are managed through this route.

There are an increasing number of acute cancer presentations that can be risk assessed for care in an emergency ambulatory setting. These include low-risk febrile neutropenia, incidental pulmonary embolism, grade 2/3 immune checkpoint inhibitor-related toxicities, such as hypophysitis, cancer-associated DVT, chemotherapy-related acute kidney injury, chemotherapy-induced nausea and vomiting, indwelling line infections, acute management of pain crises, malignant hypercalcaemia and other electrolytes abnormalities, asymptomatic brain metastases, and malignant pleural effusion.[10–13]

Ambulatory models offer the opportunity to integrate palliative and supportive care with oncology and acute services. Ambulatory enhanced supportive care models have shown utility in the management of low-risk febrile neutropenia.[14] This appears to facilitate improved access for patients to expertise in cancer care and immediate management of the complications of cancer treatment with the goal of preventing downstream complications and future emergency presentations.

The modelling of ambulatory emergency oncology services with integrated expert supportive oncology services is key for providing high quality, personalized, and sustainable emergency oncology care. It enables a greater number of patients to have their cancer complications managed at their cancer treating centre and aims to reduce attendances at overcrowded general emergency departments.

Fever in the Cancer Patient

Fever is a common acute presentation in patients with cancer second only to pain in its prevalence.[15] This can be caused by a wide range of conditions including the cancer itself, especially necrotic lesions and liver disease, pulmonary emboli, treatment-related fever (both chemotherapy and targeted therapy), G-CSF-related fever, and infective illnesses, including neutropenic sepsis.

Neutropenic Sepsis

Fever in a neutropenic patient is an acute medical emergency. Neutropenic sepsis is a potentially fatal complication of systemic anti-cancer treatment (SACT). Neutropenic sepsis is defined as a temperature >38°C and a neutrophil count <0.5×10^9/L.[16]

Most standard-dose chemotherapy regimens are associated with 6–8 days of neutropenia.[16] Neutropenic fever is observed in approximately 8 patients per 1000 receiving chemotherapy although it is recognized that a significant proportion of patients with fever post-chemotherapy do not seek medical attention.[17]

Fever during chemotherapy-induced neutropenia may be the only indication of severe infection as other signs and symptoms may be suppressed.[18] Algorithms for the management of neutropenic sepsis have been created and adapted as diagnostic and management techniques improve.

Pathophysiology of Neutropenic Sepsis

There are several contributory factors leading to the development of neutropenic sepsis including the direct effects of the chemotherapy on mucosal barriers and the immunocompromise related to the underlying malignancy. Chemotherapy-induced mucositis occurs throughout the gastro-intestinal system and seeding of the bloodstream with endogenous flora in the GI tract causes most febrile neutropenic episodes.[19]

A bacteraemia is identified in approximately 30% of patients with neutropenic sepsis.[20] Traditionally Gram-negative organisms were predominant in this cohort but the increased use of indwelling venous catheters and prophylactic antimicrobials has resulted in a higher proportion of Gram-positive organisms. Prognosis is worse in patients with proven bacteraemia with mortality rates of 18% observed in Gram-negative bacteraemia and 5% in Gram-positive bacteraemia.[20] Fungal and viral pathogens are also common in this cohort of patients. Fungal infections are typically seen in patients with prolonged neutropenia.[21]

Managing Neutropenic Sepsis

All patients with suspected neutropenic sepsis should have a thorough history and examination performed. A detailed history should include eliciting any symptoms suggestive for the focus of infection, recent exposures to infection, previous infections, establishing the chemotherapy regimen, and confirmation of antimicrobial prophylaxis. Obtaining the patient's understanding of their diagnosis and prognosis is important.

A thorough examination is required especially as signs of inflammation can be extremely subtle or absent in neutropenic patients.[16] The skin and mucous membranes should be examined carefully for erythema, cellulitis, warmth, rashes, ulcers, and evidence of mucositis. Any tunnelled lines or recent line insertion sites should be thoroughly examined for signs of infection. Any tunnelled lines or intravenous catheters should also be assessed for patency as any difficulty with withdrawing blood or infusion administration may indicate an infected clot even if the entrance site appears to have no abnormality. Patients should be questioned regarding perianal pain and examined if symptomatic.

All patients presenting with fever post-chemotherapy should have a full blood count, urea and electrolytes, liver function tests (including serum albumin), coagulation screen, C-reactive protein, lactate, and cultures performed. Obtaining cultures should not delay the initiation of antibiotic therapy.

Cerebro-spinal fluid (CSF) should be sent in those with symptoms suggestive of central nervous system infection. Many patients with malignancy and post-chemotherapy are either thrombocytopenic or coagulopathic. It is, therefore, important to correct coagulopathy or transfuse platelets prior to performing lumbar puncture.

At least two sets of blood cultures should be performed from separate venepuncture sites.[18,22,23] If the patient has a tunnelled line or central venous line in situ, a set of blood cultures should be obtained from each lumen of the line and peripherally at the same time.

Culture specimens should also be obtained from other sites as clinically indicated. Nose and throat swabs should be sent for viral pathogens including COVID-19. Sputum cultures should be sent if the patient has a productive cough. Stool cultures should be sent and evaluated for *Clostridium difficile* toxin assay. Urine culture should be sent if the patient has symptoms of a urinary tract infection or a positive urinalysis. A chest X-ray should be performed in all patients with respiratory symptoms and there should be a low threshold for performing in all patients, especially in those with a previous history of respiratory infections. Assessment for upper respiratory viral pathogens may be useful in determining the aetiology of the fever.

In solid malignancies, the presence of anatomical abnormalities is significant. Tumours that overgrow their blood supply become necrotic and infected. Different solid tumours are associated with various infections. Patients with head and neck tumours and erosion through the neck and floor of the mouth might be associated with anaerobic infection. Advanced oesophageal cancer, complicated by an obstruction, increases the risk of aspiration pneumonia. Endobronchial lung tumours are associated with chronic inflammation and recurrent post-obstructive infections.[24] Intra-abdominal tumours obstructing the genitourinary or hepato-biliary tracts could result in severe urinary tract infections or cholangitis.[25,26] Tumour invasion of the colonic mucosa might be associated with local abscess formation by enteric flora.[27] Locally advanced breast cancer is associated with an increased risk of *Staphylococcus aureus* abscess formation.[28]

Initial Management of Neutropenic Sepsis

Suspected neutropenic sepsis is an acute medical emergency and empirical antibiotic therapy should be administered immediately.[16,29–32] The goal of empirical therapy is to cover the most likely pathogens that will cause life-threatening infections in neutropenic patients. Different centres experience different patterns of frequency and resistance of causative organisms. It is essential that local microbiological guidance is followed in the choice of empirical antibiotic.

A meta-analysis comparing beta-lactam monotherapy against beta-lactam plus aminoglycoside found similar rates of survival but greater rates of morbidity and adverse events in the dual therapy group.[33] Glycopeptides, such as vancomycin, are not recommended as part of the standard initial empirical antimicrobial regimen. However, they should be considered in patients with evidence of line infection, soft tissue infection, or severe mucositis.[18]

Alongside the specific empirical antimicrobial therapy, patients with neutropenic sepsis require the same management as those with non-neutropenic sepsis ensuring adequate end-organ perfusion, early interventions, and aggressive resuscitation.[34,35]

Impeccable hand hygiene, as the most effective method of preventing the transmission of hospital infections, standard barrier precautions, and isolation in a side room are important to prevent neutropenic patients acquiring further infections.

Granulocyte colony stimulating factors (G-CSF), such as filgrastim, are not recommended as routine adjuncts to therapy in patients presenting with neutropenic sepsis.[16,36–38] Although they have been shown to reduce the duration of neutropenia and fever they have not been associated with any improved mortality outcomes.[38] There may be a small cohort of high-risk solid tumour patients where they may be of benefit and this requires careful individual patient assessment.

The use of prophylactic G-CSF decreases the incidence of FN and infection-related mortality.[39,40] Before the COVID-19 pandemic, all consensus guidelines recommended prophylactic use of G-CSF when the overall risk of neutropenic sepsis from the prescribed chemotherapy regimen is $\geq$20%.[41] Since COVID-19, guidelines recommend the expanded use of prophylactic G-CSF to include patients receiving chemotherapy regimens that have an intermediate risk of FN (>10%).[42,43] It is important that prophylactic courses of G-CSF are completed in patients presenting with fever even if they are not neutropenic. G-CSF injections can cause bone pain which should be managed with standard analgesia.

Further Management of Neutropenic Sepsis

Patients should be monitored closely with physiological observations and closely assessed for signs of infection alongside regular haematological and biochemical blood tests. The frequency of these assessments is determined by the evolving clinical picture. Changes to the initial empirical antimicrobial treatment should be guided by the evolving clinical picture and microbiological results.[16]

Patients with unexplained fever who are otherwise improving clinically should be maintained on their empirical antimicrobial therapy. If the patient continues to have fevers after 3 days of treatment the patient's septic screen should be repeated with further blood cultures and imaging based on the patient's symptoms and clinical findings.[16] The addition of further antimicrobial agents may be indicated if there are clinical suspicions of specific organisms – for example oral vancomycin if the patient has abdominal pain and diarrhoea to cover *Clostridium difficile*.[44]

Haemodynamically unstable neutropenic patients with continued fevers without a clear focus of sepsis should have their antimicrobial regimen broadened to ensure coverage of drug-resistant Gram-negative and Gram-positive organisms and anaerobes, such as extended spectrum beta-lactamases (ESBL)-producing Gram-negative bacteria and vancomycin-resistant enterococci (VRE) which are now being isolated from neutropenic patients more often than before.[16,45] Atypical infections should be considered, particularly if inflammatory markers such as C-reactive protein or procalcitonin continue to rise. CT scanning of the sinuses, chest, and abdomen is indicated to examine for evidence of abscesses or fungal infection. Empirical anti-fungal cover should be considered after 3–5 days of treatment if the patient continues to spike fevers and no focus of infection has been identified.[16,46]

Blood cultures must be taken from all lumens of tunnelled lines as part of the initial assessment. Central venous lines should not be removed as part of the initial empiric management of neutropenic sepsis.[47] However, removal of the tunnelled line is recommended in most microbiologically proven catheter-related infections with the exception of those caused by coagulase negative staphylococci.[47,48] A differential time to positivity (DTTP), which is the difference in time between positivity of results of the central line culture and the peripheral culture, of +/− 2 hours is a highly sensitive and specific indicator of a catheter-related bacteraemia.[49]

Low-Risk Febrile Neutropenia

Patients with febrile neutropenia are a heterogenous group with only a minority of treated patients developing significant medical complications.[50,51] Assessing and identifying patients who are at high or low risk for the development of severe infection and significant medical complications is important when managing patients with febrile neutropenia, as high-risk patients require hospital admission and intravenous antibiotics.[52–54]

The Multinational Association for Supportive Care in Cancer (MASCC) score is a risk scoring system for assessing and identifying patients at high and low risk of severe infection and complications.[52] The score is calculated using seven criteria associated with improved outcome. Points are accrued for each predictor. The maximum score is 26. High-risk patients have a score less than 21 and require inpatient care. Patients with a score of 21 or more have a low risk of significant complications with low rates of bacteraemia.[53]

Outpatient management of low-risk febrile neutropenia patients identified by the MASCC score is a safe and effective strategy. Caring for low-risk febrile neutropenia in an outpatient setting is proven to be safe and effective.[53–56]

Intravenous and oral antibiotic regimens have been shown to be equally effective in low-risk febrile neutropenic patients.[55,57,58] Fluoroquinolones have high oral bioavailability and a broad spectrum of activity against Gram-negative pathogens. As with high-risk patients it is important to consider local sensitivity and resistance patterns in determining the most appropriate regimen.

Outpatient management of low-risk febrile neutropenia patients has been shown to deliver cost savings alongside improving the patient experience and satisfaction.[59,60] A key component of providing outpatient ambulatory care for low-risk neutropenic patients is a clear follow-up plan and access to a 24-hour specialist oncology telephone helpline.[54] It is important that patients feel supported, know the signs and symptoms that should trigger them to seek medical assessment, and know when they should return to the hospital.

Immune Checkpoint Inhibitor Toxicity

Immune checkpoint inhibitors (ICIs) have emerged as the newest pillar of cancer treatment improving outcomes in a range of malignancies including melanoma, renal cell carcinoma, and non-small cell lung cancer.[61,62] ICIs include those targeting programmed death-1 and its ligand (PD-1 and PD-L1) and cytotoxic T lymphocyte antigen-4 (CTLA-4). Combinations of anti-PD-1/PD-L1 with anti-CTLA-4 augment immune responses and enhance clinical activity but increase the risk of toxicities.[63,64]

Immune-mediated toxicities, stemming from increased activity within the T cell lineage, range from asymptomatic or mild complications to those that are fulminant and potentially fatal. As T cells can infiltrate most tissues in the body, ICI toxicity can affect virtually any organ system.[65,66] The timing of onset of the adverse events is dependent on both the specific type of treatment and the organ system which is affected. These adverse events may be significantly delayed after initiation or completion of therapy but the majority occur within 6 months of commencing treatment.[67]

Acute presentations in patients treated with ICIs are a clinical challenge.[63,68] As symptoms may be non-specific or mimic other complications in the acutely ill cancer patient clinicians must be vigilant in diagnosing and treating immune-mediated toxicities. There are no completed prospective studies into the optimal management of immune-mediated toxicities. Guidelines for the diagnosis and management of adverse effects are based on expert opinion and consensus and are designed to minimize the impact of toxicities.[67,69]

Management of Immune Checkpoint Inhibitor Toxicities

All acutely unwell patients being treated with ICIs should undergo a comprehensive clinical work-up. There needs to be a high clinical suspicion and a low threshold for commencing appropriate therapy for immune-mediated toxicities. At the same time, they must ensure that non-immune-mediated presentations are considered and treated as these continue to form the majority in this cohort.[70,71]

The key first step in the management of immune-mediated toxicities of ICIs is recognition. Early recognition and intervention can reduce the duration and severity of the complications. The key principles of treatment include withholding the ICI drug, supporting the affected organ system, and, when necessary, initiating immune modulating medications, such as corticosteroid therapy.[63,69] The severity of the toxicity should be graded using the Common Terminology Criteria for Adverse Events (CTCAE)[72] and treatment is based on this assessment.

There is a standard approach to the management of all organ-related toxicities except for endocrinopathies. In patients experiencing severe or life-threatening toxicities supportive treatment of the affected organ system and urgent administration of high-dose intravenous corticosteroids is required. Further immunomodulating therapies are likely to be required in those with fulminant toxicity and the optimal timing of these agents remains unclear. Immune-mediated colitis will be used an example to demonstrate the approach.

Diarrhoea is a common presentation in patients on ICIs.[63,67,70] Thorough investigation for other causes of diarrhoea, especially viral and bacterial aetiologies, is necessary to facilitate appropriate treatment and ensure the immunotherapy is not discontinued erroneously. Bloody diarrhoea is an uncommon feature in immune-mediated colitis.[73] Coeliac disease and diarrhoea related to pancreatic insufficiency are rare but important immune-mediated presentations.[74] CT scan is a fast, reliable, and non-invasive modality for establishing the diagnosis of colitis.

Management of immune-mediated colitis follows the standard toxicity stepwise approach guided by CTCAE grading[67,74]:

Grade 1 (mild) – less than 4 stools a day: Supportive treatment with oral and intravenous fluids and electrolyte correction. Anti-motility agents, such as loperamide, may be used to control symptoms.

Grade 2 (moderate) – 4–6 stools a day: Supportive treatment with intravenous fluids and electrolyte correction. If symptoms persist for more than 5 days, oral prednisolone (0.5 mg/kg per 24 hr) at a tapering dose should be commenced. Steroids should tapered gradually – e.g, reducing by 10 mg every 5 days.[69,73] Colonoscopy should be considered if the diagnosis is unclear and may be useful in determining the need for more long-term immunosuppression.[74,75] Faecal calprotectin may help in distinguishing between infective and immune-mediated presentations.[76]

Grade 3/4 (severe/life-threatening) – 7 or more stools a day: High-dose methylprednisolone (1–2 mg/kg per 24 hr) should be administered and continued for an initial 3-day period alongside intravenous fluid, electrolyte replacement, and a thorough clinical work-up including a CT scan of the abdomen.[67,69,74] These patients require inpatient management.

If patients continue to experience severe diarrhoea following 3 days of high-dose steroid therapy, then infliximab (anti-TNF therapy) at a dose of 5 mg/kg should be initiated.[67,69,74,77] The use of other immunosuppressive agents, such as mycophenolate mofetil, vedolizumab and tacrolimus, should be considered in cases refractory to steroids and infliximab.[67,69,74,78] These patients require gastroenterology input.

Faecal microbiota is increasingly recognized as an important factor in the development of ICI colitis and faecal transplant is now an emerging treatment modality for severe immune-mediated colitis.[79] These are currently reserved for refractory cases, but research is being undertaken as to whether they may be utilized early in presentations and may facilitate earlier steroid weaning.

Perforation due to immune-mediated colitis is a life-threatening complication and associated with significant mortality.[80] These patients require urgent surgical review to determine the need for colectomy, intravenous antibiotics, and discontinuation of the steroids.

Acute Management of Immune-Mediated Endocrinopathies

Immune-mediated endocrinopathies include hypophysitis and diabetes mellitus presenting with diabetic ketoacidosis (DKA).[81] These can be life-threatening if not diagnosed and treated appropriately.[82–84]

Hypophysitis (inflammation of the pituitary gland) can present with either hormone defects or mass effect symptoms. Classically, hypophysitis presents with headache and fatigue. However, there are a range of non-specific symptoms including nausea, diarrhoea, malaise, and anorexia, which are common complications of cancer and other immune-mediated toxicities, that may reflect HPA axis dysfunction. Visual field defects are rare in immune-related hypophysitis.

ICI-mediated hypophysitis has two distinct patterns of disease presentation: Isolated ACTH deficiency in those treated with anti-PD-1 and PDL-1 agents and a lymphocytic hypophysitis-like condition with pituitary enlargement and multiple hormone deficiencies in those treated with anti-CTLA-4 agents.[85] These require subtle but important differences in clinical management. This illustrates the wider key point that immune-mediated toxicities of an organ system are not a single distinct entity but encompass a wider range of inflammatory pathologies. These have varying disease courses and may also require different clinical management.

Initially in patients where there is a clinical suspicion for immune-mediated hypophysitis an initial screen with cortisol, ACTH, and thyroid function should be sent. Patients should be treated with physiological doses of glucocorticosteroid (i.e., intravenous hydrocortisone 100 mg as an initial dose followed by 50 mg intravenously QDS).[82,86] Isotonic saline rather than hypertonic saline should be administered in those with significant hyponatraemia. In a retrospective analysis of 98 patients with ipilimumab-related hypophysitis those who received low-dose steroids had improved clinical outcomes both in terms of time to treatment failure, overall survival, and radiological improvement if there was pituitary swelling.[86] High-dose steroids may still be indicated in the rare presentation of hypophysitis in patients treated with CTLA-4 agents with visual field defects, cranial nerve palsies, significant pituitary enlargement, severe headache, critical illness, or significant hyponatraemia.[81,82]

In patients in whom the initial biochemistry is consistent with HPA toxicity a completed pituitary screen and MRI scan of the pituitary is necessary only in patients on CTLA-4 treatment and endocrinology referral for ongoing hormone replacement and management should be undertaken.[82]

Diabetic ketoacidosis with the classical symptoms of polyuria, polydipsia, fatigue, and weight loss is another rare but potentially life-threatening immune-mediated presentation.[87–89] These patients require standard DKA management with judicious fluid and potassium management and individualized insulin management.[81,87] These patients require long-term insulin management and diabetes support.

Immune checkpoint inhibitor toxicity management will evolve rapidly over the next decade. Many key questions including the optimal doses of corticosteroids for immune-mediated toxicity, the optimal timing of the addition of immunosuppressive agents for those with life-threatening immune-mediated toxicities, and the impact of corticosteroids on the effectiveness of ICIs need to be researched and practice adapted to findings. Clinicians working in acute oncology will not only be involved in this work but crucially in the implementation of its findings in frontline patient care.

References

1. Mansour D et al. Acute oncology service: assessing the need and its implications. *Clin Oncol* 2011;23:168–73.
2. Berger J et al. The burden of cancer on the acute medical unit. *Clin Med* 2013;13:457–9.
3. Cooksley T, Rice T. Emergency oncology: development, current position and future direction in the US and UK. *J Supportive Care Cancer* 2017;25(1):3–7.
4. National Chemotherapy Advisory Group, Chemotherapy Services in England [internet]. 2009, available at: www.dh.gov.uk/en/Publicationsandstatistics/Publications/DH_104500.
5. Ellis-Brookes L et al. Routes to diagnosis for cancer – determining the patient journey using multiple routine data sets. *Br J Cancer* 2012;7:1220–6.
6. Richardson A et al. Uncertainty and anxiety in cancer of unknown primary patient journey: a multiperspective qualitative study. *BMJ Supportive and Palliative Care.* 2015;5(4):366–72.
7. Neville-Webb H et al. The impact of a new acute oncology service in acute hospitals: experience from the Clatterbridge cancer centre and Merseyside and Cheshire cancer network. *Clin Med* 2013;13(6):565–9.
8. King J et al. Towards saving a million bed days: reducing length of stay through an acute oncology model of care for inpatients diagnosed as having cancer. *BMJ Qual Saf* 2011;20(8):718–24.
9. Lasserson DS et al. What is the evidence base for ambulatory care for acute medical illness? *Acute Med* 2018;17(3):148–53.
10. Cooksley T et al. Ambulatory emergency oncology: a key tenet for future emergency oncology care. *Int J Clin Pract* 2020;74(1):e13436.
11. Cooksley T et al. Ambulatory outpatient management of patients with low risk febrile neutropaenia. *Acute Med* 2015;14(4):178–81.
12. Hamad M, Connolly V. Ambulatory emergency care – improvement by design. *Clin Med* 2018;18(1):69–74.
13. Cooksley T et al. Immune checkpoint inhibitor-mediated hypophysitis: no place like home. *Clin Med* 2023;23(1):81–4.
14. Cooksley T et al. A novel approach to improving ambulatory outpatient management of low risk febrile neutropenia: an Enhanced Supportive Care (ESC) clinic. *Support Care Cancer* 2018;26(9):2937–40.
15. Caterino JM et al. Analysis of diagnoses, symptoms, medications and admissions among patients with cancer presenting to emergency departments. *JAMA Netw Open* 2019;2(3):e190979.
16. Klastersky J et al. Management of febrile neutropaenia: ESMO clinical practice guidelines. *Ann Oncol* 2016;27(Suppl 5):v111–18.
17. Oakley C et al. Avoidant conversations about death by clinicians cause delays in reporting of neutropenic sepsis: grounded theory study. *Psychooncology* 2017;26(10):1505–12.
18. Friefeld A et al. Clinical practice guideline for the use of antimicrobial agents in neutropenic patients with cancer: 2010 update by the infectious diseases society of America. *Clin Infect Dis* 2011;52:e56–e93.
19. Pizzo PA. Management of fever in patients with cancer and treatment-induced neutropenia. *N Eng J Med* 1993;328:1323–32.

20. Klastersky J et al. Bacteraemia in febrile neutropenic patients. *Int J Antimicrob Agents* 2007;30(Suppl 1):S51–9.
21. Ramphal R. Changes in the etiology of bacteremia in febrile neutropenic patients and the susceptibilities of the currently isolated pathogens. *Clin Infect Dis* 2004;39:S25–31.
22. Lee A et al. Detection of bloodstream infections in adults: how many blood cultures are needed? *J Clin Microbiol* 2007;45:3546–8.
23. Cockerill F et al. Optimal testing parameters for blood cultures. *Clin Infect Dis* 2004;38:1724–30.
24. Chrysikos S et al. Endobronchial metastasis from renal cell carcinoma as a reason for recurrent pulmonary infections. *Adv Respir Med* 2018;86(5):245–8.
25. Zhang GQ et al. Outcomes of preoperative endoscopic nasobiliary drainage and endoscopic retrograde biliary drainage for malignant distal biliary obstruction prior to pancreaticoduodenectomy. *World J Gastroenterol* 2017;23(29):5386–94.
26. Smit LC et al. Infectious complications after major abdominal cancer surgery: in search of improvable risk factors. *Surg Infect (Larchmt)* 2016;17(6):683–93.
27. Klaver CEL et al. Postoperative abdominal infections after resection of T4 colon cancer increase the risk of intra-abdominal recurrence. *Eur J Surg Oncol* 2018;44(12):1880–8.
28. Cilekar M et al. An atypical cause of rapidly progressing breast lump with abscess formation: pure squamous cell carcinoma of the breast. *J Cancer Res Ther* 2015;11(4):1023.
29. Flowers C et al. Antimicrobial prophylaxis and outpatient management of fever and neutropenia in adults treated for malignancy: American Society of Clinical Oncology clinical practice guideline. *J Clin Onc* 2013;31:794.
30. Rosa R, Goldani L. Cohort study of the impact of time to antibiotic administration on mortality in patients with febrile neutropenia. *Antimicrob Agents Chemother* 2014;58(7):3799–803.
31. Perron T et al. Time to antibiotics and outcomes in cancer patients with febrile neutropenia. *BMC Health Serv Res* 2014;14:162.
32. Mattison G et al. A nurse-led protocol improves the time to first dose intravenous antibiotics in septic patients post chemotherapy. *Support Care Cancer* 2016;24(12):5001–5.
33. Paul M et al. Beta-lactam versus beta-lactam-aminoglycoside combination therapy in cancer patients with neutropaenia. *Cochrane Database Syst Rev* 2003: CD003038.
34. Angus D, van der Poll T. Severe sepsis and septic shock. *N Engl J Med* 2013;369:840–51.
35. Dellinger R et al. Surviving sepsis campaign: international guidelines for management of severe sepsis and septic shock: 2012. *Crit Care Med* 2013;41(2):580–637.
36. Garcia-Carbonero R et al. Granulocyte colony-stimulating factor in the treatment of high risk febrile neutropenia: a multicentre randomized trial. *J Natl Cancer Inst* 2001;93:31–8.
37. Clark O et al. Colony-stimulating factors for chemotherapy-induced febrile neutropenia: a meta-analysis of randomised controlled trials. *J Clin Onc* 2005;23:4198–214.
38. NICE Guideline CG151. Neutropenic sepsis: prevention and management of neutropenic sepsis in cancer patients [internet], 2012; available at: https://www.nice.org.uk/guidance/cg151.
39. Cooper K et al. Granulocyte colony-stimulating factors for febrile neutropenia prophylaxis following chemotherapy: systematic review and meta-analysis. *BMC Cancer* 2011;11:404.
40. Cooksley T et al. Emerging challenges in the evaluation of fever in cancer patients at risk of febrile neutropenia in the era of COVID-19: a MASCC position paper. *Support Care Cancer* 2021;29(2):1129–138.
41. Smith TJ et al. Recommendations for the use of WBC growth factors: American Society of Clinical Oncology clinical practice guideline update. *J Clin Oncol* 2015;33(28):3199–212.
42. ESMO, Supportive care strategies during the COVID-19 pandemic [internet], available at: https://www.esmo.org/guidelines/cancer-patient-management-during-the-covid-19-pandemic/supportive-care-in-the-covid-19-era.
43. ASCO, COVID-19 patient care information [internet], available at: https://www.asco.org/asco-coronavirus-information/care-individuals-cancer-during-covid-19.
44. Ligova A et al. Clostridium difficile associated diarrhoea – problem of oncological patient? *Klin Onkol* 2009;22:108–16.

45. Moghnieh R et al. Third generation cephalosporin resistant Enterobacteriaceae and multi-drug resistant gram-negative bacteria causing bacteremia in febrile neutropenia adult cancer patients in Lebanon, broad spectrum antibiotics use as a major risk factor and correlation with poor prognosis. *Front Cell Infect Microbiol* 2015;5:11.

46. Kibbler C. Empirical antifungal therapy in febrile neutropenic patients: current status. *Curr Top Med Mycol* 1997;8:5–14.

47. Mermel LA et al. Clinical practice guidelines for the diagnosis and management of intravascular catheter related infection. *Clin Infect Dis* 2009;**49**:1–45.

48. Raad I et al. Management of the catheter in documented catheter-related coagulase-negative staphylococcal bacteremia: remove or retain? *Clin Infect Dis* 2009;49:1187–194.

49. Krause R et al. Detection of catheter related bloodstream infections by the differential time to positivity method and Gram-stain-acridine orange leukocyte cytospin test in neutropenic patients after hematopoietic stem cell transplantation. *J Clin Microbiol* 2004;42:4835–7.

50. Paesmans M et al. Predicting febrile neutropenic patients at low risk using the MASCC score: does bacteremia matter? *Support Care Cancer* 2011;19:1001–8.

51. Lynn J et al. Risk factors associated with complications in patients with chemotherapy-induced febrile neutropenia in emergency department. *Hematol Oncol* 2013;31:189–96.

52. Klastersky J et al. The multinational association for supportive care in cancer risk index: a multinational scoring system for identifying low-risk febrile neutropenic cancer patients. *J Clin Onc* 2000;18:3038–51.

53. Klastersky J, Paesmans M. The Multinational Association for Supportive Care in Cancer (MASCC) risk score: 10 years of use for identifying low risk neutropenic cancer patients. *Support Care Cancer* 2013;21:1487–95.

54. Cooksley T et al. Ambulatory outpatient management of patients with low risk febrile neutropaenia. *Acute Med* 2015;14(4):178–81.

55. Klastersky J et al. Outpatient oral antibiotics for febrile neutropenic cancer patients using a score predictive for complications. *J Clin Oncol* 2006;24:4129–34.

56. Elting L et al. Outcomes and cost of outpatient or inpatient management of 712 patients with febrile neutropenia. *J Clin Onc* 2008;26:606–11.

57. Freifeld A et al. A double-blind comparison of empirical oral and intravenous antibiotic therapy for low-risk febrile patients with neutropenia during cancer with chemotherapy. *N Engl J Med* 1999;341:305–11.

58. Kern W et al. Oral antibiotics for fever in low-risk neutropenic patients with cancer: a double-blind, randomized, multicentre trial comparing single daily moxifloxacin with twice daily ciprofloxacin plus amoxicillin/clavulanic acid combination therapy – EORTC infectious diseases group trial XV. *J Clin Onc* 2013;31:1149–56.

59. Teuffel O et al. Cost-effectiveness of outpatient treatment for febrile neutropenia in adult cancer patients. *Br J Cancer* 2011;104:1377–83.

60. Teuffel O et al. Health-related quality of life anticipated with different management strategies for febrile neutropenia in adult cancer patients. *Support Care Cancer* 2012;20:2755–64.

61. Ribas A, Wolchok JD. Cancer immunotherapy using checkpoint blockade. *Science* 2018;359:1350–5.

62. Johnson DB et al. Immune checkpoint inhibitor toxicity in 2018. *JAMA* 2018;320(16):1702–3.

63. Postow MA et al. Immune-related adverse events associated with immune checkpoint blockade. *N Engl J Med* 2018;378:158–68.

64. Wang DY et al. Fatal toxic effects associated with immune checkpoint inhibitors: a systematic review and meta-analysis. *JAMA Oncol* 2018;4(12):1721–8.

65. Naidoo J et al. Toxicities of the anti-PD-1 and anti-PD-L1 immune checkpoint antibodies. *Ann Oncol* 2015;26:2375–91.

66. Knight T et al. Acute oncology care: a narrative review of the acute management of neutropenic sepsis and immune-related toxicities of checkpoint inhibitors. *Eur J Intern Med* 2017;45:59–65.

67. Haanen J et al. Management of toxicities from immunotherapy: ESMO clinical practice guidelines for diagnosis, treatment and follow up. *Ann Oncol* 2017;28:iv119–42.

68. Webb P et al. Problem-based review: immune-mediated complications of "checkpoint inhibitors" for the acute Physician. *Acute Med* 2017;16(1):21–4.

69. Brahmer JR et al. Management of immune-related adverse events in patients treated with immune checkpoint inhibitor therapy: American Society of Clinical Oncology clinical practice guideline. *J Clin Onc* 2018;17:1714–68.

70. El Majzoub I et al. Adverse effects of immune checkpoint therapy in cancer patients visiting the emergency department of a comprehensive cancer center. *Ann Emerg Med* 2019;73(1):79–87.

71. Cooksley T et al. Emergency presentations in patients treated with immune checkpoint inhibitors. *Eur J Cancer* 2020;130:193–7.

72. US Dept of Health and Human Services. Common Terminology Criteria for Adverse Events; Version 5.0 [internet], 2014, available at: https://ctep.cancer.gov/protocoldevelopment/electronic_applications/docs/ctcae_v5_quick_reference_5x7.pdf).

73. Wang Y et al. Immune-checkpoint inhibitor-induced diarrhea and colitis in patients with advanced malignancies: retrospective review at MD Anderson. *J ImmunoTherapy Cancer.* 2018;6(1):37.

74. Dougan M et al. Multinational Association of Supportive Care in Cancer (MASCC) 2020 clinical practice recommendations for the management of severe gastrointestinal and hepatic toxicities from checkpoint inhibitors. *Support Care Cancer* 2020;28(12):6129–43.

75. Wang Y et al. Endoscopic and histologic features of immune checkpoint inhibitor-related colitis. *Inflamm Bowel Dis* 2018;24:1695–705.

76. Reddy HG et al. Immune checkpoint inhibitor-associated colitis and hepatitis. *Clin Transl Gastroenterol* 2018;9:180.

77. Johnson DH et al. Infliximab associated with faster symptom resolution compared with corticosteroids alone for the management of immune-related enterocolitis. *J Immunother Cancer* 2018;6:103.

78. Abu-Sbeih H et al. Outcomes of vedolizumab therapy in patients with immune checkpoint inhibitor-induced colitis: a multi-center study. *J Immunother Cancer* 2018;6:142.

79. Wang Y et al. Fecal microbiota transplantation for refractory immune checkpoint inhibitor-associated colitis. *Nat Med* 2018;24(12):1804–8.

80. Eggermont A et al. Adjuvant ipilumumab versus placebo after complete resection of high risk stage III melanoma: a randomised controlled trial. *Lancet Oncol* 2015;16:522–30.

81. Girotra M et al. The current understanding of the endocrine effects from immune checkpoint inhibitors and recommendations for management. *JNCI Cancer Spectr* 2018;2(3):21.

82. Higham C et al. Society for endocrinology endocrine emergency guidance: acute management of the endocrine complications of checkpoint inhibitor therapy. *Endocrine Connections* 2018;7(7):G1–G7.

83. Ryder M et al. Endocrine-related adverse events following ipilimumab in patients with advanced melanoma: a comprehensive retrospective review from a single institution. *Endocrine-Related Cancer* 2014;21:371–81.

84. Joshi M et al. Hypophysitis: diagnosis and treatment. *Eur J Endocrinol* 2018;179:R151–63.

85. Percik R et al. Diagnostic criteria and proposed management of immune-related endocrinopathies following immune checkpoint inhibitor therapy for cancer. *Endocr Connect* 2023;12(5):e220513.

86. Faje A et al. High-dose glucocorticoids for the treatment of ipilimumab-induced hypophysitis is associated with reduced survival in patients with melanoma. *Cancer* 2018;124(18):3706–14.

87. Chang LS et al. Endocrine toxicity of cancer immunotherapy targeting immune checkpoints. *Endocr Rev* 2019;40(1):17–65.

88. Perdigoto AL et al. Checkpoint inhibitor-induced insulin-dependent diabetes: an emerging syndrome. *Lancet Diabetes Endocrinol* 2019;S2213–8587(19)30072–5.

89. Stamatouli AM et al. Collateral damage: insulin dependent diabetes induced with checkpoint inhibitors. *Diabetes* 2018;67:1471–80.

3

Pain and Symptom Management

3A

Pain Assessment

Dan Monnery, Joanne Collins, Lesley Howells, and Jennifer Vidrine

The management of pain in cancer is increasingly complex. New treatments are leading to emergent treatment-related pain syndromes, whilst an expanding population of cancer survivors requires expertise in the management of pain in a post-cancer cohort. Even in incurable cancer, patients are living longer, giving new concern to the use of strong opioids. Whilst common in the palliative setting, strong opioids have time-dependent risks and toxicities which need to be taken into account from the first prescription. Practices which are commonplace need to be critically reviewed.

What Does a Good Pain Assessment Look Like?

Your assessment should include a review of the patient history and appropriate investigations, including:

- Is there a lesion (new or known) causing pain in this area?
- Does the change in pain represent a change in the cancer or a treatment toxicity?
- What medications are feasible in light of the patient's tolerance, allergies, and hepatic/renal clearance?

Reversing any underlying cause is important if possible: Often, treatment with anticancer therapies can help pain control.

There are a number of different 'pain syndromes' in cancer; that is, clusters of symptoms and descriptors which may help you to determine the cause and most appropriate course of treatment. Whilst these are not all fully understood and new pain syndromes are emerging all the time, Table 3A.1 gives a synopsis of those commonly encountered current and potential treatment strategies.

DOI: 10.1201/9781003369912-5

TABLE 3A.1

Cancer-Related Pain Syndromes

Pain Syndrome	Symptoms/Descriptors	Potential Treatments
Localized tumour pain	• Located around area of tumour • If located in the skin or muscle the pain is well localized and 'sharper' (described as 'somatic') whereas if in the viscera the pain is dull and more poorly localized (described as 'visceral') • Often described as a throbbing sensation and worsened by anything which distorts or puts pressure on the area	• Opioids (more effective in somatic than visceral pain) • NSAIDs or COX 2 inhibitors • Steroids • Nefopam • Radiotherapy • Systemic anticancer therapy • Nerve block
Neuropathic pain	• Resulting from tumour compressing nerves (including spinal cord compression) resulting in radiculopathy (pain follows a nerve root) OR glove and stocking distribution of pain from a systemic cause (chemotherapy, diabetes, vitamin B12 deficiency, paraneoplastic) • Regardless of anatomical location pain is often described as shooting or burning • Often has associated cardinal features such as numbness, paraesthesia, dysaesthesia, and allodynia • Commonly worse at night	• Gabapentinoid • Amitriptyline • Duloxetine • Steroids (if taking pressure off a compressed nerve or spinal cord) • Lidocaine plasters (if superficial) • Consider clonazepam • Capsaicin (for peripheral neuropathy) • Radiotherapy (if taking pressure off a compressed nerve or spinal cord) • Nerve block
Bone pain	• Localized over site of bone lesion (e.g. tumour of pathological fracture) • Pain is dull at rest, sharp and severe on movement • Affects movement of the affected area or inability to weight bear	• NSAIDs or COX 2 inhibitors • Opioids (often pre-movement) • Bisphosphonates (especially for breast and prostate malignancies and myeloma) • Surgery • Radiotherapy • Nerve block
Coeliac plexus pain	• Associated with tumours which can compress the coeliac plexus or cause coeliac nodal disease e.g. pancreatic, gastric, and cholangiocarcinomas • Dull 'gnawing' epigastric pain • Constant but can be relieved by leaning forwards • Can feel like a tight band around the upper abdomen and back; on occasion the pain can be predominantly in the back	• Combinations of opioids and neuropathic agents • Consider nerve block (coeliac plexus block) early • Steroids • NSAIDs or COX 2 inhibitors • May require more complex medications, e.g. ketamine or methadone

(Continued)

TABLE 3A.1 (CONTINUED)

Cancer-Related Pain Syndromes

Pain Syndrome	Symptoms/Descriptors	Potential Treatments
Retroperitoneal nodal pain	• Associated with tumours which cause retroperitoneal spread e.g. colon, gynaecological, sarcoma, germ cell • Dull ache in the back • Can be worse on standing and associated with a 'dragging' sensation in the back, relieved by lying down	• Combinations of opioids and neuropathic agents • Steroids • NSAIDs or COX 2 inhibitors • May require more complex medications, e.g. ketamine or methadone
Psoas syndrome	• Associated with tumours which compress or irritate the psoas muscles, e.g. renal or those which can metastasize to the psoas muscles or surrounding area, e.g. breast, melanoma • No pain at rest, then severe back pain when getting up and walking • Pain relieved again when sitting down • Pain radiates from hip to groin on the affected side • Pain can be worse at night if legs are straight and can be relieved by propping a pillow under the knee on the affected side	• Muscle relaxants: Pridinol, baclofen, benzodiazepines • Clonazepam • Combinations of opioids and neuropathic agents • Steroids • NSAIDs or COX 2 inhibitors • Radiotherapy • May require more complex medications, e.g. ketamine or methadone
Chemotherapy-induced peripheral neuropathy	• Glove and stocking distribution of neuropathic pain occurring following chemotherapy such as taxanes and platinum-based chemotherapy • Regardless of anatomical location pain is often described as shooting or burning • Often has associated cardinal features such as numbness, paraesthesia, dysaesthesia, and allodynia • Sometimes associated with other systemic features of neuropathy e.g. delayed gastric emptying, postural hypotension	• Duloxetine[1] • Venlafaxine • Amitriptyline/nortriptyline • Capsaicin • If associated spasm, muscle relaxants: Pridinol, baclofen, benzodiazepines • Physiotherapy for desensitization and exercises
Mucositis pain	• Resulting from radiotherapy or chemotherapy and affecting any area of mucosa; commonly mucositis affecting oral and oesophageal areas causes pain • Associated with visual changes to the mucosa including redness, ulceration, and bleeding • Pain can affect the ability to eat and drink • Saliva may feel thick and unable to swallow	• Topical morphine 0.2% mouthwash[2] • Topical benzydamine (do not swallow) • Caphosol • Oxetacaine and antacid • Systemic opioids
Treatment-related arthralgias	• Symmetrical polyarthropathy which can affect any joints • Induced commonly by aromatase inhibitors (in breast cancer) but also noted with immunotherapies and androgen blockage in prostate cancer (enzalutamide and bicalutamide)	• Duloxetine • Prednisolone 20 mg daily for 1 week, then 10 mg daily for 4 weeks, then 5 mg daily for 1 week, then stop (in immunotherapy induced) • NSAIDs/COX 2 inhibitors • Occasionally low-dose gabapentinoids can help

(Continued)

TABLE 3A.1 (CONTINUED)

Cancer-Related Pain Syndromes

Pain Syndrome	Symptoms/Descriptors	Potential Treatments
Myofascial pain	• Focal pain surrounding an area of injury or tumour associated with muscle tension or spasm • Can be triggered by neuropathy leading to muscle spasm • Commonly associated with areas of point tenderness or hardness over muscle	• Muscle relaxants: Pridinol, baclofen, benzodiazepines • Lidocaine plasters if superficial • Acupressure/acupuncture • Trigger point injections • Physiotherapy
Rectal pain	• Commonly associated with tumours of the anorectal canal or radiation involving the rectum • Sharp internal pain, feels like 'hot poker' • Can radiate to lower back, anterior abdomen, and upper legs • Associated with tenesmus • Commonly worse on sitting, relieved by lying down	• Nifedipine, diltiazem, or baclofen if tenesmus • Gabapentinoid • Amitriptyline • Duloxetine • Steroids (prednisolone suppositories or enemas or systemic steroids) • Opioids • May require more complex medications, e.g. ketamine or methadone • Consider defunctioning colostomy • Consider nerve block
Post-radiation neuropathy	• Occurs during or post-radiotherapy • Associated with radiation along the affect nerve distribution – this may be trigeminal neuropathy in head and neck radiotherapy or rib radiculopathy in breast radiotherapy for example • Regardless of anatomical location pain is often described as shooting or burning • Often has associated cardinal features such as numbness, paraesthesia, dysaesthesia, and allodynia • Commonly worse at night	• Gabapentinoid • Amitriptyline • Duloxetine • Lidocaine plasters (if superficial)
Total pain	• Occurs in the absence of a biological explanation of the pain; is in excess of what can be expected from a biological injury • Not responsive to escalating doses of opioids • Commonly associated with high levels of patient and family distress and/or complex psychosocial factors	• Psychological interventions • SSRIs • Benzodiazepines (low dose, short course) • Physiotherapy/occupational therapy for functional rehabilitation • Consider chronic pain approach and referral

Remember that pain cannot always be classified exactly as it is above. Some patients will have more than one pain syndrome and your treatment will need to encompass all aspects – remembering to focus on patient tolerance, goals, and any sensitivities or cautions to individuals or combinations of medications.

The Multinational Association for Supportive Care in Cancer has some guidance on the management of some pain syndromes but at the time of writing these are still emerging and research is ongoing, so managing these complex situations is largely based on clinical judgement.

Why Use a Tool?

Pain measurement tools vary from numeric rating scales (from 0 to 10) to more detailed scales looking to determine the type of pain e.g. the Leeds Assessment for Neuropathic Symptoms and Signs (LANSS).[3] If a tool is used it should be patient-reported so that the actual experience of the patient is captured. Furthermore, tools which capture multimodal experience of pain (including wellbeing, e.g. the Edmonton Symptom Assessment Scale, ESAS[4]) may be preferred. For patients with cognitive or communication difficulties, observation of pain-related behaviour and discomfort is advocated;[5] however additional tools which can be used to help assessment in this group of people include the Abbey pain scale for patients with advanced dementia.[6]

Pharmacological Treatment of Pain

In terms of analgesic choice, it is important to consider the patient's medical and drug history, their stage of illness, and their current systemic anticancer treatment (SACT) regimen, and analgesic preferences. You should also consider up to date blood results to ensure adequate metabolism and excretion of certain drugs. Not all analgesics work for all types of pain so your pain history may help you to classify the pain to determine which analgesia is most appropriate.

i. *NSAIDs*

Non-steroidal anti-inflammatory drugs work in cancer pain by reducing peripheral nociceptor stimulation by prostaglandins and prevent the central action of prostaglandins in facilitating sensitization. They are useful in inflammatory pains such as arthrlagias, myalgias, and post-surgical pain but given the pro-inflammatory nature of tumours and their metastases, they can also be useful for tumour pain and bone metastases; arguably they could be used more in cancer pain on an individual patient basis.[7] Caution should be given to prescribing them in impaired renal function or those with a bleeding risk and they are contraindicated in patients with brittle asthma, where a COX 2 inhibitor should be considered instead. They require ongoing monitoring of renal function. The risks of GI ulceration and renal impairment are higher with prolonged use. Caution is required when prescribing NSAIDs and COX 2 inhibitors in patients receiving SACT, and they should be avoided in patients who are receiving or have recently received nephrotoxic chemotherapy.

ii. *Neuropathic Agents*

Neuropathic agents reduce the sensitivity of damaged nerves to generating action potentials or prevent the transmission of neurotransmitters in the spine. They are useful in neuropathic pain but can also be useful where there is a neuropathic component to a more complex pain such as coeliac plexus or pelvic pain. The usual first-line neuropathic agent would be either a low dose of a tricyclic antidepressant, such as amitriptyline, or a gabapentinoid such as pregabalin or gabapentin.[8] Amitriptyline is sedating and may help improve sleep; however it has anticholinergic adverse effects which many patients are unable to tolerate. Duloxetine is an alternative for the management of neuropathic pain[8] and is preferred in some centres. The dose should be titrated to effect with regular review to ensure the patient is taking it correctly and deriving benefit.

If pain still persists at night, it may be appropriate to consider a short course of a benzodiazepine, such as clonazepam which has both anxiolytic and muscle relaxant properties and is reported to improve both cancer-related and non-cancer-related neuropathic pain in selected patients.[9]

iii. *Opioids*

Opioids are a useful tool in the management of acute pain; however in the chronic setting opioids carry a significant risk of toxicity, tolerance, and addiction. Traditionally in the palliative setting, opioids have been used with relative freedom due to the poor prognoses negating the need to consider long-term toxicities. However, the improved prognoses afforded by new treatments mean the use of opioids needs a rapid rethink.

iv. *Opioids in the Palliative Setting*

For patients with palliative cancer and prognoses of less than 18 months, opioids remain a viable option for management of pain. In those patients approaching end of life, opioids have versatility in how they can be administered and are widely effective and overall well tolerated for time-limited periods. They tend to be more effective in nociceptive pain than neuropathic pain.[10] but can nevertheless serve as a useful adjunct in other pain types whilst more appropriate medications are being titrated to therapeutic levels. Whilst previously prescribed in accordance with the World Health Organization analgesic ladder, it is now thought the weak opioids (codeine/tramadol) contribute little benefit and significant side effects when used as part of cancer pain management so are not advised. Instead, patients should have early access to strong opioids. A combination of instant-release and slow-release formulations is often used to control pain over a 24-hour period, the aim being to escalate the slow-release dose gradually and safely to a level where a patient requires 2 or fewer breakthrough doses in any 24-hour period.[9] Instant-release oral opioids such as morphine and oxycodone liquid can take an hour to reach peak plasma concentration.[11, 12], so patients should be permitted to use these early if they feel pain 'breaking through' and should keep a record of use to enable the clinician to adjust the background dose accordingly. Due consideration should be given to the patient's blood results as renal and/or liver impairment will affect the choice of opioid which is appropriate for the patient.

v. *Opioids in the Chronic Setting*

This includes patients who have treatable but not curable cancer with prognoses of greater than 18 months, and those who have received curative treatment but are left with long-term pain resulting either from the cancer or its treatment. Whilst opioids are not completely contraindicated, you should be clear when starting them how long their use is to be continued and consideration given to other options if longer term management is needed.

There is little evidence of benefit of long-term opioids in the chronic setting with regards to pain, quality of life, or functioning.[13] Furthermore, existing pain guidelines advising the use of opioids in cancer pain management are more applicable to the palliative setting than the survivorship setting. High-dose opioid therapy carries a risk of dependence and opioid-related mortality.[14] Buprenorphine however may be appropriate in the management of chronic cancer and non-cancer pain.[15] Preliminary data suggest that compared to morphine and other opioids, buprenorphine causes less hyperalgesia and tolerance, and has less effect on the immune and endocrine systems.[15] As buprenorphine is less constipating than morphine, has a better long-term safety profile, and is considered safe in renal impairment,[9] it may be preferred for those with longer prognoses and pain requiring opioid management.

vi. *Interventional Pain Approaches*

Interventional pain approaches should not be overlooked in the management of cancer pain and can often avoid the need for escalating levels of analgesia with an unfavourable risk/benefit ratio. Whilst certain interventions such as cordotomies should only be provided to those with limited prognoses, others can be well tolerated over a longer period (e.g. intrathecal pump). Early consideration should be given to referral to pain teams and interventional anaesthetists for consideration of interventions in patients whose prognosis is a caution to medications with long-term toxicities.[16]

vii. *Patient Information*

Medicines associated with dependence include benzodiazepines, opioids, and gabapentinoids. These medicines can provide lasting symptom management with a favourable balance of benefits and adverse effects for many people. But like all medicines, they do not work for everyone and can have negative consequences that outweigh their benefits, especially long term. Prior to prescribing any medicines associated with dependence, you should discuss treatment options with the patient so they can make informed decisions about their care.[17] Drug driving advice is also a requirement by law and patients must be advised not to drive if they are affected by their medication.[18]

viii. *Non-Pharmacological Treatment of Pain*

Non-drug treatments often complement prescribed analgesia. Pain often leads to functional impairment; therefore it is important to explore this with patients and refer to local services such as physiotherapy and occupational therapy which can help with functional pain management and rehabilitation. Gentle exercise should be encouraged where possible. Non-weight bearing exercise such as swimming[19] can be useful for improving muscle strength and fatigue whilst minimizing pain; however individualized, expert advice is valuable in long-term pain management.

Responding to Psychosocial Needs

Psychological distress from a cancer diagnosis can have a big impact on health and wellbeing and in turn affect the patient's experience of pain. The gate control theory of pain[20] describes the physiological mechanisms by which psychology can influence pain, occasionally leading to a state of 'total pain'. Stress, worry, anger, anxiety, and emotional hypervigilant states can all influence pain and may require a range of input including further information, peer support, formal or informal counselling, psychological therapies, or medications.

Responding to psychosocial needs is essential in pain management. Advances in 'Third Wave Cognitive Behavioural Therapy (CBT)' and meaning-based existential psychotherapeutic approaches mean there is growing evidence for the successful use of psychological interventions. These include formal and informal, group, couple, and individual therapies which have been shown to improve patients' experiences of pain.[21,22] Furthermore, these therapies support patients in living meaningfully with uncertainty,[23] fear of recurrence and progression,[24] and anticipatory grief.[25] In particular, Acceptance and Commitment Therapy (ACT) is a trans-diagnostic and trans-contextual psychological approach for people living with the pain of advanced cancer and is recommended to help patients live the quality of life that is meaningful to them despite pain. You can access these through referral to NHS psycho-oncology services and third sector resources such as Maggie's.[26] These services will also help with relationship concerns, including helping patients clarify and rehearse constructive conversations with family, colleagues, and employers.

Health behaviour models stress that a person's motivation to accept help is enhanced by a respected figure (you), making relevant and achievable suggestions, and offering role models with similar stories.[27] Patients are more likely to access psychoeducational resources and websites to help with problems like intimacy,[28] talking with children,[29] or financial and employment worries,[30] if you suggest them. Also, they are more likely to access psychological support if you tell them how others have benefitted.[31] See further Box 3A.1.

BOX 3A.1 KEY CONSIDERATIONS IN CANCER PAIN ASSESSMENT

- What type of pain is it? Does it fit with a cancer-related pain syndrome?
- Is this pain explained by known disease or is further investigation needed?
- Do blood results, comorbidities, and other medications contraindicate any analgesics?
- How does the pain impact the patient's ability to function?
- How does the pain affect their mood and relationships and what support mechanisms do they have?
- What goals do they have – what changes will you see in their lifestyle from better pain management?

BOX 3A.2   KEY CONSIDERATIONS WHEN PRESCRIBING ANALGESIA

- Is this medication suitable for the type of pain?
- Are there any contraindications based on past medical history, blood results, or other medications including concurrent SACT?
- How long will the patient need the medication? Are there safer alternatives for longer term pain control if needed?
- Is early involvement of interventional pain approach indicated?
- Who will oversee this medication long term, and if there will be a need to reduce it after a period, whose responsibility is this?
- What does this patient need to know about this medication to keep them safe and are there other medications they should avoid in future?

Long-Term Care

Shared decision making is a fundamental part of ensuring the success of any management plan. Patient reported outcome measures (PROMs) can be a valuable way of patients being able to monitor their pain and other symptoms and then feedback responses and trends to their healthcare teams. The value of empowering and equipping patients with the tools, language, and opportunities to be involved in all decision making about their care cannot be overstated.

Increasingly, with patients receiving treatment which confers an improved prognosis, it is imperative that treatment plans are arrived at considering the length of time that they may need to continue for and any potential interaction with current or future medications. See further Box 3A.2.

Any interventions used should be regularly reviewed to ensure that they are still necessary, appropriate, tolerated, and effective. General practitioners and other key members of the community care team should be kept fully involved with support instigated by secondary or tertiary care with clear agreement as to who is overseeing which element of care and where to seek support.

Consider the broad spectrum of support that is available from other services. Chronic pain clinics, outpatient therapies, and third sector organizations all offer emotional and practical support which can be transformative in the management of pain. These services often have access to a specialized Multidisciplinary Team (MDT) with expertise in managing issues around pain, although there is national variation in where these services are available and how to access them and not all have expertise in the management of cancer pain. There is an increasing array of published and virtual resources available for those living with cancer pain[32] and a number of online forums for those with lived experience of pain to receive peer support. Patients can find huge benefit in being able to speak and relate to others going through similar situations.

References

1. Loprinzi CL et al. Prevention and management of chemotherapy-induced peripheral neuropathy in survivors of adult cancers: ASCO guideline update. *J Clin Oncol.* 2020;38(28):3325–3348.

2. Saunders DP et al. Systematic review of antimicrobials, mucosal coating agents, anesthetics, and analgesics for the management of oral mucositis in cancer patients and clinical practice guidelines. *Support Care Cancer.* 2020;28(5):2473–2484.

3. Bennett M. The LANSS pain scale: the Leeds assessment of neuropathic symptoms and signs. *Pain.* 2001;92(1–2):147–1457.

4. Bruera E et al. The Edmonton symptom assessment system (ESAS): a simple method for the assessment of palliative care patients. *J Palliat Care.* 1991;7:6–9.

5. Fallon M et al. Management of cancer pain in adult patients: ESMO clinical practice guidelines. *Ann Oncol.* 2018;29(Suppl 4):iv166–iv191.

6. Abbey J et al. The abbey pain scale: a 1-minute numerical indicator for people with end-stage dementia. *Int J Palliat Nurs.* 2004;10(1):6–13.

7. Schüchen RH et al. Systematic review and meta-analysis on non-opioid analgesics in palliative medicine. *J Cachexia Sarcopenia Muscle.* 2018;9(7):1235–1254.

8. National Institute for Health and Care Excellence. Neuropathic pain – pharmacological management, CG173 [internet], 2013, updated 2020, available at: https://www.nice.org.uk/guidance/cg173/evidence/full-guideline-pdf-4840898221.

9. Twycross R et al., *Palliative Care Formulary (PCF 8).* 8th ed. Nottingham: Palliativedrugs.com Ltd; 2022.

10. Chahl LA. Opioids – mechanisms of action. *Aust Prescr.* 1996;19:63:5.

11. Glare PA, Walsh TD. Clinical pharmacokinetics of morphine. *Ther Drug Monit.* 1991;13(1):1–23.

12. Kinnunen M et al. Updated clinical pharmacokinetics and pharmacodynamics of oxycodone. *Clin Pharmacokinet.* 2019;58(6):705–725.

13. Faculty of Pain Medicine of the Royal College of Anaesthetists. Opioids aware [internet], available at: https://www.fpm.ac.uk/opioids-aware (accessed Jan 2023).

14. Oxford University Hospitals NHS Foundation Trust. Resources for GPs regarding opioids and chronic pain. For GPs: opioids and chronic pain [internet], 2023, available at https://www.ouh.nhs.uk/services/referrals/pain/opioids-chronic-pain.aspx#! (accessed Jan 23).

15. Foster B et al. Buprenorphine. *J Pain Symptom Manage.* 2013;45(5):939–949.

16. Gulia A et al. Impact of early intervention in pain management in cancer patients: a randomized controlled study in a tertiary care cancer hospital. *Clin J Pain.* 2021;1;37(4):259–264.

17. National Institute for Health and Care Excellence. Medicines associated with dependence or withdrawal symptoms: safe prescribing and withdrawal management for adults, NG215 [internet], 2022, available at www.nice.org.uk/guidance/ng215.

18. Department for Transport, Drug Driving and Medicine. Advice for healthcare professionals, drug driving and medicine: advice for healthcare professionals [internet], 2014, available at: https://www.gov.uk/government/publications/drug-driving-and-medicine-advice-for-health care-professionals (accessed Jan 2023).

19. NHS, Ways to Manage Chronic Pain [internet], 2021, available as https://www.nhs.uk/live-well/pain/ways-to-manage-chronic-pain/ (accessed Jan 2023).

20. Melzack R, Wall PD. Pain mechanisms: a new theory. *Science.* 1965;150:971–979.

21. Cosio D, Demyan A. Behavioral medicine: how to utilize acceptance and commitment therapy in primary care. *Pract Pain Manag.* 2021;21(2).

22. Winger JG et al. Meaning-centered pain coping skills training: a pilot feasibility trial of a psychosocial pain management intervention for patients with advanced cancer. *J Palliat Med.* 2022;25(1):60–69.

23. Fang P et al. Effectiveness of acceptance and commitment therapy for people with advanced cancer: a systematic review and meta-analysis of randomized controlled trials. *J Advanced Nursing* 2023;79(2):519–538.

24. Bergerot CD et al. Fear of cancer recurrence or progression: what is it and what can we do about it? [internet]. *Am Soc Clin Oncol Educ Book.* 2022:42, 18–27, available at: https://ascopubs .org/doi/10.1200/EDBK_100031.

25. Butow P et al. Editorial: uncertainty, anxiety, and fear of cancer recurrence. *Front Psychol.* 2021;12:811602.

26. Maggie's, Cancer support, available at: https://www.maggies.org/cancer-support/ (accessed Feb 2023).

27. Ajzen I. The theory of planned behaviour: reactions and reflections. *Psychol. Health.* 2011;26(9):1113–1127.

28. Cancer Council NSW. Sexuality, Intimacy and Cancer [internet], 2021, available at: https:// www.cancercouncil.com.au/cancer-information/managing-cancer-side-effects/sexuality -intimacy/ (accessed Feb 2023).

29. Fruitfly Collective. Building new ways to support children, adults and families affected by cancer [internet], available at: https://www.fruitflycollective.com/ (accessed Feb 2023).

30. Maggie's, Help with money worries, current and future employment, and employability [internet], available at: https://www.maggies.org/cancer-support/our-support/help-money -worries/ (accessed Feb 2023).

31. Scherrens A-L et al. Using behavioral theories to study health-promoting behaviors in pallia- tive care research. *Palliative Medicine.* 2023;37(3):402–412.

32. Cancer Research UK, Resources and Support for Cancer Pain [internet], 2021, available at: https://www.cancerresearchuk.org/about-cancer/coping/physically/cancer-and-pain-control /resources-and-support (accessed Feb 2023).

3B

Symptom Management

Charlotte Leach, Jo Thompson, and Ashique Ahamed

Introduction

As the number of anti-cancer treatments expands and patients live with cancer through-out different treatments, a flexible and dynamic approach to symptom management is required. This chapter will explore the management of common physical symptoms which arise from the cancer or following therapies, and consider how supportive oncology clinicians will need to adapt their management depending on overall goals of care and disease trajectory.

Long-Term Effects of Opioids

There is no set definition of long-term use of opioid therapy, but many studies define "long-term" use as >90 days. Presently, there is no consensus for the diagnosis and management of opioid-induced endocrinopathies, bone health, so-called narcotic bowel syndrome, and other consequences of long-term opioids.

i. *Hypogonadism*

The most recognized endocrinopathy is hypogonadism. This is caused by a decrease in the pulsatile release of gonadotrophin-releasing hormone from the hypothalamus, which in turn decreases the release of LH and FSH from the anterior pituitary. LH and FSH directly stimulate the gonads to release testosterone from the testes (and the ovaries to a lesser extent), or estradiol and progesterone from the ovaries. The effects of opioid-induced hypogonadism are diverse, and may have a significant impact on quality of life; for example, reduced libido, menstrual cycle changes, erectile dysfunction, and depression.

The severity of hypogonadism is directly proportional to the dose and type of opioid and is reversible upon stopping opioids.[1] Tapentadol and buprenorphine are associated with a lower degree of hypogonadism, and in particular, buprenorphine exerts minimal effect on sex hormones.[2] This is encouraging and may be used to inform shared decision making with patients when discussing benefits and harms of long-term opioid therapy. For males who continue with long-term opioid therapy, androgen replacement with transdermal testosterone (patches or gel) may be considered, although is not common practice

DOI: 10.1201/9781003369912-6

within supportive care settings in the UK. The role of sex hormone replacement (oestrogen, progesterone, or testosterone) in females is unknown.

Supportive care clinicians must consider the risk of hypogonadism when caring for patients receiving opioid therapy. Given the growing range of endocrine adverse effects from opioid therapy, but also from immunotherapy and steroid-induced hyperglycaemia, collaboration with endocrine and andrology specialist colleagues would be a welcome addition to the supportive oncology team. The practical arrangements for the creation of an effective supportive oncology Multidisciplinary Team (MDT) are discussed in Chapter 9.

ii. *Bone Health*

Opioids cause reduced bone density via both a direct effect through impairing osteoblastic activity, and an indirect effect through reduced sex hormone production from hypogonadism.[3] A meta-analysis of 30 studies involving people aged >65 years showed an association between opioid therapy and falls, injuries, and fractures, with an effect size ranging from 0.15 to 0.71. Furthermore, those who used higher doses of opioids appeared to have a higher risk of fracture.[4]

Given the increased risks of falls, fractures, and death following a hospital admission for a bony fracture, supportive oncology clinicians face several unanswered questions regarding how to identify, risk stratify, and optimize bone health in those patients receiving long-term opioids. Arguably, many patients have several additional risk factors for fractures as sequalae of cancer or anti-cancer treatment such as bony metastases, use of glucocorticoids, and treatment that can precipitate menopause (i.e., oophorectomy) and some chemotherapies or aromatase inhibitors that suppress ovarian function.

Whilst publications such as the 'European Society of Medical Oncology Clinical Practice Guidelines on Bone Health in Cancer' focus on prevention and management of skeletal-related events, there is an absence of any evidence or recommendations for the optimization of bone health in patients receiving long-term opioid therapy.[5]

As the specialty of supportive oncology evolves, important questions regarding the optimization of bone health for patients receiving long-term opioid therapy will require close consideration and research; for example, is there a role for screening patients at higher risk of bone fracture, and which (if any) patients should be offered bone-targeted therapies such as bisphosphonates?

iii. *Narcotic Bowel Syndrome*

Narcotic bowel syndrome is another significant long-term effect of opioid therapy, which often presents with regular and worsening abdominal pain in the context of long-term opioid therapy. The exact pathophysiology is unknown, although chronic opioid-induced hyperalgesia is one of the likely mechanisms. It is clinically diagnosed and can be very challenging to manage as the cornerstone of treatment is opioid cessation.

Temporal Trends

There is evidence that a reduction in temporal trends of opioid prescribing by both oncologists and non-oncologists (20.7% and 22.8% respectively) was accompanied by a 15%

increase over four years in opioid prescribing by palliative care physicians.[6] This is attributed to many factors including changes in opioid prescribing legislation and increased use of non-opioid analgesics such as gabapentin.

It is important to not overlook the implication that patients with cancer may be adversely affected by the recommendations to reduce opioid therapy directed at chronic non-cancer pain.

Mitigating the Risks of Long-Term Opioid Therapy

If opioids are ineffective or no longer indicated, opioid dose tapering is an obvious approach to management. However, the absence of research exploring harms, benefits, and practicalities of opioid tapering in cancer populations leaves supportive oncology clinicians navigating unchartered waters.

Opioid dose tapering may not be appropriate for all patients. Some patients living with chronic pain due to cancer or anti-cancer treatment (such as post thoracotomy pain, radiation-induced necrosis) may require long-term opioid therapy to achieve a satisfactory quality of life.

Supportive oncology clinicians must also be mindful to balance the pressure to reduce opioid prescribing in response to public health recommendations against the potential to cause physical and psychological harm from inadequately managed cancer pain. In response to the "opioid epidemic" and concerns that restrictive legislation was denying patients with cancer-appropriate access to opioid therapy, the American Society of Clinical Oncology (ASCO) produced a Policy Statement.[7] This recognizes the heterogeneity and complexities of cancer pain and asserts that patients with cancer pain should be considered as a special population in the context of the public health approach to the "opioid epidemic".

Presently, there are no guidelines for opioid dose tapering in patients with cancer pain. Shared decision making and honest discussions about the goals, harms, and benefits of opioid dose tapering (particularly so with concurrent benzodiazepine administration) are essential.

Given the nuances and complexities of balancing the harms and benefits of opioid dose tapering in the supportive care population, collaboration, expert opinion, and research are long overdue. Indeed, will supportive oncology clinicians adopt a similar approach to opioid dose tapering as chronic pain clinicians, or respond to the growing call to recognize the heterogeneity and complexity of needs for those receiving supportive care through developing evidence-based, consensus recommendations?

Neurological Complications

Cancer and cancer therapies can damage both the central and the peripheral nervous systems. Prominent targets include the brain, resulting in cognitive impairment, neuro-endocrine dysfunction, depression, and anxiety; and the peripheral nerves resulting in neuropathy. The area of neurological complications has gained growing attention within cancer research but there are still limitations in some areas including neurological complications relating to CAR-T therapy (which include tremors), problems with attention and expressive language, disorientation, and short-term memory. Complications can occur a few days after treatment and generally resolve quickly. However, further study is warranted relating to longer term outcomes which are currently poorly understood.[8] More detail relating to common complications is given below.

i. *Chemotherapy-Induced Peripheral Neuropathy (CIPN)*

CIPN is the most prevalent neurological complication of chemotherapy.[9] It occurs predominantly due to the damage to sensory peripheral nerves (although motor and autonomic deficits can be a feature) by some oral or intravenous anti-tumour agents. CIPN causes debilitating symptoms which can affect physical function resulting in a negative impact on quality of life.[10]

The most common agents causing CIPN are platinum drugs (oxaliplatin, cisplatin), taxanes (paclitaxel, docetaxel), vincristine, bortezomib, thalidomide, and eribulin. Approximately 68% of patients experience CIPN (from any form of chemotherapy drug) 1 month after treatment, 60% at 3 months, and 30% at 6 months or longer.[11] Patients commonly describe a symmetrical sensory neuropathy in the hands and feet – known as a 'glove and stocking' distribution.

Management of the symptom relies on early identification and comprehensive assessment. This is challenging as not only do patients find it difficult to describe their symptoms but they may also be experiencing multiple other issues and see CIPN symptoms as a low priority to discuss. There is also a reluctance to report due to the fear this will result in chemotherapy being reduced or stopped.[12]

Management options are limited, the mainstay being delaying, reducing, or stopping the causative agent. Duloxetine, a serotonin noradrenalin reuptake inhibitor (SNRI), has been shown to reduce pain associated with CIPN and is currently the only recommended pharmaceutical treatment.[13] Studies with small numbers of participants have shown some benefit with high-dose (179 mg) capsaicin patches; however, this requires specialist advice and assessment.[9] There is emerging evidence that some exercise programmes focusing on endurance, strength, balance, and resistance are beneficial.[14] Exercise programmes have focused both on prevention and rehabilitation in relation to the impact of CIPN symptoms on quality of life. Studies have highlighted that adherence to exercise programmes has been an issue, suggesting motivating patients may be challenging. Education and information given at the start and throughout treatment with the aim of increasing patients' familiarity with CIPN is vital.[15] This in turn can lead to more timely reporting of the symptoms supporting improved assessment and joint management decisions between patients and clinicians.

ii. *Metastatic Spinal Cord Compression (MSCC)*

MSCC refers to compression of the spinal cord due to direct pressure secondary to the extension of the tumour, or metastatic spread, causing spinal collapse or instability. This in turn threatens (or causes) neurological disability.[16]

Patients most at risk are those with lung, breast, or prostate cancers, myeloma, and lymphoma. Improved cancer treatments mean more patients with metastatic disease are living longer putting them at risk of developing spinal metastases and thus the potential to develop MSCC.

Treatment includes urgent radiotherapy, steroids, and sometimes surgery with the aim being for patients to maintain a degree of mobility – patients are suddenly faced with the prospect of paraplegia with a permanent reduction of independence alongside the acknowledgement their disease has progressed.[17] Outcomes are very much dependent on functional status at diagnosis and prompt treatment.

Of equal importance from a functional perspective is the assessment and management of bowel and bladder function.[18] Whilst care delivered by nurses and other health care professionals is attentive to these needs, promoting self-management is sometimes overlooked.[19] Many patients are catheterized on initial diagnosis but for some, intermittent self-catheterization after radiotherapy should be considered.[16] Individualized care surrounding bowel management should be planned. Following assessment and consideration of patient preferences this could involve dietary advice, stool softeners and stimulants, or regimens involving constipating agents and digital rectal evacuation.[20]

Giving patients the opportunity to discuss their individualized goals should also be an urgent priority at diagnosis of MSCC. Rehabilitation is important but will result in long periods of time in hospital. For individuals with a short prognosis, this may not be in line with their personal preferences and priorities.[18]

iii. *Seizures*

Seizures represent a serious and potentially life-threatening complication for people with cancer. The most common cause is intracranial disease with an estimated 29–60% of people with primary brain tumours and 10–40% of people with intracranial metastatic disease experiencing seizures.[21] Seizures have major consequences for patients physically, socially, and emotionally. They carry an increased risk of sudden death[22] and mental health disorders such as anxiety and depression;[23] they also mean patients can no longer drive.[24]

Health care professionals (HCPs) have a significant role to play in supporting patients to manage their seizures and reducing the negative impact on their quality of life (QoL). Treatment involves ascertaining the underlying cause, treating the cause where possible, and, when indicated, initiating antiepileptic drugs (AEDs). Whilst it used to be common practice, the use of AEDs prophylactically for people with intracranial disease is no longer recommended.[25]

The overarching goal of treatment plans is to obtain seizure control with acceptable safety and tolerability of AED.[23] Unfortunately, whilst seizures can be effectively treated and prevented with AEDs, they are associated with numerous potential adverse effects such as somnolence, rash, weight changes, cognitive dysfunction, teratogenicity, anxiety, and emotional lability.[26] These side effects can in turn have a negative impact on QoL, the risk being that patients find them intolerable and either do not comply with the prescribed regimen or stop taking them altogether putting them at risk of further life-threatening seizures.[26]

The challenge for HCPs is to review seizure management along with supporting patients and giving them the confidence to report side effects so these can be monitored. Where possible, monotherapy with AEDs is preferable.[21] because patients taking only one drug report "a better view" of their health.

Gastrointestinal Symptoms

Gastrointestinal (GI) symptoms are a common complication of the disease. These symptoms can be caused by the primary tumour, as well as by cancer treatment.

It is estimated that up to 90% of patients with advanced cancer experience at least one GI symptom. The commonly reported symptoms include nausea, vomiting, diarrhoea, constipation, and anorexia. These symptoms can have a significant impact on the patient's QoL and can lead to hospitalization and increased health care costs.

The mechanisms underlying GI symptoms in cancer patients are often multifactorial:

- Biochemical: Cytotoxic drugs, opioids, hypercalcemia, infection.
- Delayed gastric emptying: Autonomic dysfunction, paraneoplastic syndromes, opioids.
- Gastrointestinal: Bowel obstruction, cytotoxic drugs, radiation colitis, constipation, and post-transplant mucositis.
- Cranial and vestibular: Raised intracranial pressure from cerebral metastasis, primary brain tumour, bleed, etc.
- Psychosocial: Anticipatory nausea, general anxiety.

The Multinational Association of Supportive Care in Cancer (MASCC) recommends the following antiemetics in the management of nausea and vomiting in advanced cancer:[27]

- First line: Metoclopramide or haloperidol.
- Second line: Methotrimeprazine (levomepromazine) or olanzapine.

i. *Chemotherapy-Induced Nausea and Vomiting (CINV)*

CINV can affect up to 80% of patients receiving highly emetogenic chemotherapy (HEC) and up to 30% of patients receiving moderately emetogenic chemotherapy (MEC). The management of CINV involves a combination of prophylactic and rescue therapies and supportive care measures, with the goal of preventing or treating CINV as early and effectively as possible.

Supportive oncology clinicians should also note these general principles around the management of nausea and vomiting:

- Reverse what is reversible including hypercalcemia, constipation, and opioid-induced bowel dysfunction.
- Review potential adverse effects and tolerability to various antiemetics on an individual basis and select route (PO/parenteral) of administration based on severity of symptoms. Some patients may require a temporary subcutaneous syringe pump infusion to help with severe symptoms.

The current guidelines recommend the use of 5-HT3 receptor antagonists (i.e., palonosetron), NK-1 receptor antagonists (i.e., aprepitant), and corticosteroids for the prevention of CINV. Olanzapine (atypical antipsychotic with antagonistic activity at dopamine, serotonin, histamine, and acetylcholine receptors) is recommended for the prevention of emesis in highly and moderately emetogenic chemotherapy regimens, as well as treatment of refractory CINV. Benzodiazepines can be helpful in mitigating anticipatory nausea.[28] Non-pharmacological interventions such as acupuncture, acupressure, and cognitive-behavioural therapy can also be used as adjunctive therapies for the management of CINV.

ii. *Malignant Bowel Obstruction (MBO)*

MBO is estimated to occur in 10–28% of patients with gastrointestinal cancers and up to 51% of patients with advanced ovarian cancer. The cause of MBO can be either mechanical or functional in nature. Mechanical obstruction can either be due to extrinsic compression of the intestinal lumen from omental masses and adhesions or intraluminal obstruction by growing tumour in the bowel. Functional obstruction arises from motility disorders due to tumour infiltration of mesentery, nerve and/or coeliac and enteric plexus and para-neoplastic syndromes.[29] Other factors that can contribute to MBO include drugs such as opioids, constipation, and fibrosis.

   MBO can cause nausea, vomiting, and pain. Often management is conservative. In cases of complete bowel obstruction, the patient should be kept nil by mouth with adequate provision for IV hydration and NG tube insertion in cases of recurrent high-volume vomiting. A short-term trial of parenteral dexamethasone (dose range 4 mg to 16 mg/24 hrs) can reduce periluminal inflammation and help with the symptoms.[30] Anti-secretory agents (i.e., hyoscine butylbromide, and somatostatin analogues) can reduce the volume of vomitus. Metoclopramide can be used in cases of partial bowel obstruction but should be stopped if it exacerbates pain or if the obstruction worsens.

iii. **Constipation**

Around 40–90% of patients with cancer suffer from constipation due to a variety of causes. This includes:

- Drugs: Opioids, tricyclic antidepressants, anticholinergics, antiemetics (cyclizine, 5HT3 antagonists) certain chemotherapy regimens.
- Biochemical: Hypercalcemia, hypokalaemia, dehydration, hypothyroidism.
- Neurological: Autonomic dysfunction, spinal tumours.
- Mechanical: Abdominal or pelvic mass, peritoneal carcinomatosis.
- Diet: Low fibre intake, anorexia, poor food and fluid intakes.
- Lack of privacy or need for assistance during toileting.

Principles for management of constipation:

- Reverse treatable causes e.g., hydration, correction of electrolyte imbalance. Reduce polypharmacy where possible.
- Lifestyle modifications: Encourage activity and physical mobility, encourage oral intake of fluids, regular review of bowel habits.
- A combination of stimulant laxatives (i.e. senna, sodium picosulphate) and osmotic or stool softeners (i.e. docusate sodium) can help relieve constipation. In

some cases, patients may require rectal intervention including suppositories and enemas.

iv. *Opioid-Induced Constipation (OIC)*

Opioids cause constipation by binding to μ-opioid receptors in the GI tract, which reduces GI secretions, increases colonic fluid reabsorption, and increases anal sphincter tone. Typically, OIC causes hard, dry stool, resulting in straining.

OIC is commonly under-diagnosed and under-treated, leading to significant impact on QoL. A thorough assessment is essential, including asking how the bowel habit may have changed since starting opioid therapy. Supportive oncology clinicians should bear in mind that tramadol and transdermal fentanyl and buprenorphine are less constipating.[31]

Conventional laxatives are often ineffective in resolving OIC. Peripherally acting opioid antagonists (PAMORAs) – either given separately or combined with the opioid – reverse OIC without compromising the opioid analgesic effect or causing withdrawal and should be considered in all patients receiving opioid therapy.[32]

v. *Pelvic Radiation Disease (PRD)*

Radiotherapy for pelvic malignancy can encompass healthy tissue. This can lead to a range of GI toxicities to the irradiated area. Up to half of patients undergoing pelvic radiotherapy can suffer from PRD. PRD is discussed further in Chapter 4B.

vi. *Chemotherapy-Induced Diarrhoea*

A range of chemotherapy agents and newer treatments including immunotherapy and targeted therapy can result in diarrhoea.

Management of diarrhoea involves active hydration and replacement of electrolytes. Constipating agents such as loperamide may be used once infective causes and colitis have been excluded. Severe immunotherapy-related colitis may occasionally require high-dose steroids.

vii. *Cancer Treatment and the Gut Microbiome*

The gut microbiome is a complex ecosystem of bacteria, viruses, and fungi that play a vital role in maintaining gut health. Chemotherapy drugs can disrupt the balance of the gut microbiome, leading to an overgrowth of pathogenic bacteria and a decrease in beneficial bacteria. Chemotherapy-induced gut dysbiosis can lead to an imbalance in the gut microbiome, contributing to diarrhoea, constipation, and other GI symptoms.

There is also increasing evidence that the stability and imbalances of the gut microbiome may have an impact on the growth of tumours and on the efficacy of anti-cancer treatments, such as immunotherapy. The science is new but emerging treatments for restoring a healthy gut microbiome include dietary modifications, use of probiotic nutrients, and faecal transplantation[33]

Oral Symptoms

i. *Oral Mucositis (OM)*

Oral mucositis is a common complication of cancer treatment affecting 40% of patients receiving standard doses of chemotherapy and 100% of patients receiving high-dose chemotherapy i.e., with haematopoietic stem cell transplants and head and neck radiotherapy.[34] Severity ranges from mild erythema to severe ulceration, bleeding, and infection. This can result in treatment delays or discontinuation, poor nutrition, increased requirement for opioid analgesics, and hospitalization.

The challenge for supportive oncology clinicians is the lack of predictive factors for those most at risk. This is well-recognized and current research is focusing on understanding individual risk factors to support the provision of personalized care.[35] Female sex, advancing age, excessive alcohol intake, and smoking status appear to be indicators for those at increased risk.

Key elements of care include pain relief, dietary support, and infection prevention.[36] To this end, oncology centres need oral care protocols in place that include a validated assessment tool (for example, the common terminology criteria for adverse events, CTCAE[37]) and management guidelines. There is growing interest in the use of intraoral photobiomodulation (low-level laser therapy) for prevention of oral mucositis in patients receiving chemo-radiotherapy for head and neck cancers.[38] MASCC and the International Society for Oral Oncology (ISOO) produced updated guidelines for the management of mucositis secondary to cancer therapy.[38]

The guideline highlights basic oral care as important for all patients receiving SACT and radiotherapy to the head and neck region, including:

- A focus on the importance of regular oral care and enhanced compliance,
- The regular use of bland rinses (saline, sodium bicarbonate) to assist in oral clearance.

ii. *Salivary Gland Hypofunction and Xerostomia*

Salivary gland hypofunction (SGH) refers to a reduced salivary flow rate and xerostomia refers to patient reported subjective sensation of dry mouth. Saliva has a vital role to play in tooth integrity, cleansing of the oral cavity, oral comfort, prevention of infections, swallowing, and speech.[38]

SGH affects 100% of patients having head and neck radiotherapy, the effects being permanent. It is not surprising that SGH has a profound impact on patients physically (pain, discomfort, infections), emotionally (embarrassment, frustration), and socially (impact on speech and eating). The response is to support patients holistically and encourage good, regular oral hygiene whilst recognizing that motivation may be low due to the intense nature of treatment.

iii. *Taste Dysfunction*

Taste dysfunction is a complication of cancer and cancer treatment; the effects can be permanent having a detrimental effect on nutritional status. Taste disturbances can affect the desire to eat and enjoyment of food which in turn affects patients emotionally and socially. The involvement of dietitians at an early stage is recommended.

Other strategies involve enhancing the taste of food with salt/sugar and other flavourings but also paying attention to other aspects of flavour such as presentation, smell, consistency, and temperature.[39] There is evidence from one small RCT to suggest tetrahydrocannabinol (THC) may be useful in taste alterations;[40] however, further evidence is needed to support routine recommendation.

iv. *Oral Candidiasis*

Oral candidiasis can develop because of cancer (specifically due to the impact on performance status meaning oral hygiene may be more difficult), and cancer-related treatments such as steroids, immunosuppression, systemic antibiotics, systemic anti-cancer therapy, and radiotherapy (causing mucosal damage and xerostomia).

Good oral assessment is important and where possible treatment of the underlying cause i.e., xerostomia. Topical and systemic medications are available for treating the infection; topical agents (i.e., miconazole gel) are appropriate for localized infection, and systemic medications (i.e., fluconazole) are used for more serious or widespread infections affecting the oro-pharynx, for example.

References

1. Fountas A et al. Opioid-induced endocrinopathies. *Lancet Diabetes Endocrinol* 2020;8:68–80.
2. Davis M. Twelve reasons for considering buprenorphine as a frontline analgesic in the management of pain. *Support Oncol* 2012;10:2009–219.
3. Coluzzi F et al. The unsolved case of bone-impairing analgesics: the endocrine effects of opioids on bone metabolism. *Ther Clin Risk Management* 2015;11:515–523.
4. Yoshikawa A et al. Opioid use and the risk of falls, falls injuries and fractures among older adults: a systematic review and meta-analysis. *J Gerontol A Biol Sci Med Sci* 2020;75(10):1989–1995.
5. Coleman R et al. on behalf of the ESMO guidelines committee: bone health in cancer: clinical practice guidelines. *Ann Oncol* 2020;31 (12):1650–1663.
6. Jairam V al. Temporal trends in opioid prescribing patterns among oncologists in the medicare population. *J Natl Cancer Inst* 2021;113(3):274–281.
7. American Society of Clinical Oncology, ASCO Policy Statement on Opioid Therapy: Protecting Access to Treatment for Cancer-Related Pain [internet], 2016, available at: https://www.asco .org/sites/new-www.asco.org/files/content-files/advocacy-and-policy/documents/2016 -ASCO-Policy-Statement-Opioid-Therapy.pdf (accessed Jan 2023).
8. Tallantyre E et al. Neurological updates: neurological complications of CAR T therapy. *J Neurol* 2021;268:1544–1554.
9. Maihofner C et al. Chemotherapy induced peripheral neuropathy (CIPN): current therapies and topical treatments with high concentration capsaicin. *Supportive Care in Cancer* 2021;29:4223–4238.
10. Tanay M et al. The experience of chemotherapy-induced peripheral neuropathy in adult cancer patients: a qualitative thematic synthesis. *Eur J Cancer Care* 2017;26:e12443.
11. Seretny M et al. Incidence, prevalence and predictors of chemotherapy-induced peripheral neuropathy: a systematic review and meta-analysis. *Pain* 2014;155(12):2461–2470.

12. Salgado T et al. Reporting of paclitaxel induced peripheral neuropathy symptoms to clinicians among women with breast cancer: a qualitative study. *Supportive Care in Cancer* 2020;28:4163–4172.

13. Loprinzi C et al. Prevention and management of chemotherapy-induced peripheral neuropathy in survivors of adult cancers: ASCO guideline update. *J Clin Oncol* 2020;38(28):3325–3348.

14. Tanay M et al. A systematic review of behavioural and exercise interventions for the prevention and management of chemotherapy-induced peripheral neuropathy symptoms. *J Cancer Survivorship* 2021;17(1):254–277.

15. Tanay M et al. Clinician and patient experiences when providing and receiving information and support for managing chemotherapy-induced peripheral neuropathy: a qualitative multiple-methods study. *Eur J Cancer Care* 2021;31:e135178.

16. National Institute for Health and Care Excellence, Spinal metastases and metastatic spinal cord compression, guideline 234 [internet], 2023, available at: https://www.nice.org.uk/guidance/ng234 (accessed Sept 2023).

17. Harris M. Quality of life in patients with malignant spinal cord compression: a review of evidence-based literature. *Int J Palliative Nursing* 2016;22(1):37–43.

18. Troke R, Andrewes T. Nursing considerations for supporting cancer patients with metastatic spinal cord compression: a literature review. *Br J Nursing* 2019;28(17):S24–S29.

19. Warnock C et al. Evaluating the care of patients with malignant spinal cord compression at a regional cancer centre. *Int J Palliative Nursing* 2008;14(10):510–515.

20. National Institute for Health and Care Excellence, Faecal Incontinence in Adults: Management [internet], 2007, available at: https://www.nice.org.uk/guidance/cg49 (accessed Dec 2021).

21. Castro N, Milligan T. Seizures in patients with cancer. *Cancer* 2020;126:1379–1389.

22. National Institute for Health and Care Excellence, Epilepsies in children, young people and adults [internet], 2022, available at https://www.nice.org.uk/guidance/ng217 (accessed Dec 2022).

23. Weller M et al. Epilepsy meets cancer: when, why and what to do about it? *Lancet Oncol* 2012;13:375–82.

24. Driver Vehicle and Licensing Agency (DVLA) Epilepsy and Driving [internet], available at: https://www.gov.uk/epilepsy-and-driving.

25. Chang S et al. Anticonvulsant prophylaxis and steroid use in adults with metastatic brain tumours: summary of SNO and ASCO endorsement of the congress of neurological surgeon's guidelines. *Neuro-Oncology* 2019;21(4):424–427.

26. Monsour M et al. Antiepileptic drugs in the management of cerebral metastases. *Neurosurgical Clin N Am* 2020;31(4):589–601.

27. Davis M et al. MASCC antiemetics in advanced cancer updated guideline. *Support Care Cancer* 2021;29(12):8097–8107.

28. National Comprehensive Cancer Network. *Antiemesis*. NCCN Clinical Practice Guidelines in Oncology (NCCN Guidelines®). Version 2.2020 (accessed Mar 2023).

29. Cousins SE et al. Surgery for the resolution of symptoms in malignant bowel obstruction in advanced gynaecological and gastrointestinal cancer. *Cochrane Database Syst Rev* 2016;2016(1):CD002764.

30. Madariaga A et al. MASCC multidisciplinary evidence-based recommendations for the management of malignant bowel obstruction in advanced cancer. *Support Care Cancer* 2022;30(6):4711–4728.

31. Davies A et al. Opioid-induced constipation in patients with cancer: a "real-world," multicentre, observational study of diagnostic criteria and clinical features. *Pain* 2021;162(1):309–318.

32. Davies A et al. MASCC recommendations on the management of constipation in patients with advanced cancer. *Support Care Cancer* 2020;28(1):23–33.

33. Lee KA et al. The gut microbiome: what the oncologist ought to know. *Br J Cancer* 2021;125:1197–1209.

34. Gibson RJ et al. Systematic review of agents for the management of gastrointestinal mucositis in cancer patients. *Supportive Care in Cancer* 2013;21:313–326.

35. Wardill H et al. Prediction of mucositis risk secondary to cancer therapy: a systematic review of current evidence and call to action. *Supportive Care in Cancer* 2020;28:5059–5073.
36. Elad S et al. MASCC/ISOO clinical practice guidelines for the management of mucositis secondary to cancer therapy. *Cancer* 2020;4423–4431.
37. US Department of Health and Human Services. Common Terminology Criteria for Adverse Events v.5 [internet], 2017, available at: https://evs.nci.nih.gov/ftp1/CTCAE/CTCAE_4.03/Archive/CTCAE_4.0_2009-05-29_QuickReference_8.5x11.pdf (accessed Feb 2023).
38. Mercadante, V et al. Salivary gland hypofunction and/or xerostomia induced by nonsurgical cancer therapies: ISOO/MASCC/ASCO guideline. *J Clin Oncol* 2021;39(25):2825–2843.
39. Jones J et al. MASCC / ISOO expert opinion on the management of oral problems in patients with advanced cancer. *Supportive Care in Cancer* 2022;30:8761–8773.
40. Brisbois T et al. Delta-9-tetrahydrocannabinol may palliate altered chemosensory perception in cancer patients: results of a randomised, double-blind, placebo-controlled pilot trial. *Ann Oncol* 2011;22:2086–2093.

3C

Cancer-Associated Thrombosis

Simon Noble

Introduction

The aim of this chapter is to give those involved in supportive oncology a practical approach to cancer-associated thrombosis (CAT).

The recommendations here should be viewed as a general guide and should not replace local policy or guidelines. Prescribing should follow local licencing legislation and dosing. But questions remain surrounding the clinical usefulness of some existing guidelines. Do they offer real insight into the management of patients in the 'real world'? Have unrealistic inclusion/exclusion criteria and the lack of research validation through randomized control trials limited their real-world effectiveness? Perhaps further reflections into the nature and management of common concerns can help supportive oncology teams improve clinical practices in this area.

An understanding of the pathophysiology of CAT, pharmacodynamics of anticoagulants within the context of cancer, multimorbidity, and polypharmacy is essential and should be used as part of a multidisciplinary team approach to deliver patient-centred care. Such care should take into consideration the values and preference of each individual, which will differ according to their own personal experiences and understanding of the condition.

Background to Clotting

Clotting (or coagulation as it is more correctly known), is a normal part of the body's healing process. Without a clotting system, simple cuts or bruises would continue to bleed.

Venous clots comprise predominantly of erythrocytes, held together by a mesh of fibrin. Platelets also feature, usually the first responders to endothelial damage, and are later embedded within the fibrin structure where they are believed to play a role in clot contraction. As good as the body is at forming blood clots, it is equally effective at removing them through the process of fibrinolysis; plasmin, acting like scissors, nibbling away at away at the thrombus until it is removed.

Initially, clots form an unstable jelly-like structure, with further layers laid down if the prothrombotic tendency continues. This is when it is at its most unstable and at greatest risk of breaking off and embolizing. Over time, particularly in the presence of anticoagulants,

DOI: 10.1201/9781003369912-7

the clot will adhere to the endothelial wall, contract, and stabilize. The risk of pulmonary emboli is subsequently reduced, and ensuing fibrinolysis will limit the clot burden as the body's hemostatic system breaks down and resorbs the material.

The first five to seven days are usually when the incipient clot is at its most unstable. Once a patient has been anticoagulated past this point, the clot is less likely to break off and embolize. It usually takes six weeks for a clot to be considered stable enough to withstand an interruption of anticoagulation. This is important when considering a pre-surgical patient, who has been found to have an incidental thrombus.

Risk Factors for Developing Cancer-Associated Thrombosis (CAT)

The annual incidence of VTE in the general population is approximately 0.1%, most usually precipitated by a transient risk factor such as immobility, surgery, or an acute inflammatory illness.

Virchov's Triad[1] divides the main risk factors for developing venous thromboembolism (VTE) into:

  i. Endothelial damage
  ii. Stasis
  iii. Hypercoagulability

However, this is an oversimplification. It is rarely one factor that leads to a clot forming. There are several risk factors which increases risk, including increasing age, obesity, and inherited thrombophilia.

Cancer patients are at particular risk of developing VTE. The cancer itself induces a hypercoagulable state through the direct release of procoagulants and by the release of proinflammatory molecules such as cytokines and interleukins. The risk of cancer is further increased by disease progression – metastatic disease conferring a further 20-fold increase in risk. Similarly anticancer treatments such as surgery, radiotherapy, brachytherapy, and systemic anticancer treatments are all independent risk factors which will add to the overall prothrombotic state.[2]

The thrombogenicity of the cancer also varies according to the primary. The most prothrombotic cancers are primary brain, haematological (e.g., myeloma), pancreatic, and lung. Breast and prostate cancer are less thrombogenic but since they are such common cancers and continue to receive systemic anticancer therapies (SACT) for metastatic disease, they form a significant number of CAT diagnoses.

Presentation of VTE

The classic presentation of deep vein thrombosis (DVT) comprises of a swollen, tender erythematous leg – yet in real life such a triad of symptoms is rarely seen. Most commonly patients will give a history of limb pain, often in the back of the calf. This, particularly with unilateral leg swelling should provoke a high index of suspicion for DVT.

Similarly, the textbook presentation of pulmonary embolus (PE) with sudden onset dyspnoea, chest pain, and haemoptysis, festooned with the S1Q3T3 ECG changes, is seldom seen and unrepresentative of the majority of PE presentations.

The presentation of PE will depend upon the thrombotic load of the pulmonary embolus (or emboli if more than one is present). Small PEs may have minimal (if any) symptoms. Larger emboli will manifest as dyspnoea with associated chest pain. Emboli which are too large to embolize beyond the main pulmonary arteries may cause profound dyspnoea and cardiovascular collapse.

Patients have historically described delays in their VTE being diagnosed, despite presenting with corresponding symptoms. This is usually because they are attributed to pathologies other than VTE.[3] Dyspnoea for example is a common symptom which is also caused by other common cancer-associated pathologies such as infection, pulmonary metastases, pleural effusion, anaemia, etc., which are often considered rather than a PE. Likewise, leg swelling is commonly encountered with hypoalbuminaemia or when local lymphadenopathy obstructs lymphatic and/or venous flow. Similarly, swelling and erythema may be diagnosed as cellulitis instead of DVT.

It is important to recognize that cancer-associated pathology and comorbidities do not exist in isolation; it is quite normal for patients to have cellulitis and DVT. Likewise, a breathless patient can be anaemic and have a pleural effusion and pulmonary emboli at the same time.

Finally, do not dismiss a diagnosis of VTE on the basis of absent symptoms. In particular, the likelihood of dyspnoea being due to a PE is in no way lessened by the absence of DVT signs or symptoms. Data suggest 80% of pulmonary emboli are diagnosed in the absence of DVT symptoms.

Diagnosis

In usual clinical practice, radiology requests are unlikely to be entertained without a positive D-dimer test. However, they are unhelpful in the evaluation of a cancer patient. D-dimers are specific cross-linked fibrin derivatives, produced following the degradation of fibrin by plasmin.[4] Concentrations are therefore raised by thrombolysis, making them a highly sensitive indicator for VTE. They are a useful exclusory test for of VTE, with a negative predictive value of close to 100%. However, their utility in the cancer setting is limited because despite a high sensitivity for VTE, they have a low specificity since levels may be raised following either recent surgery, liver disease, cancer, pregnancy, and/or infection. D-dimers are therefore not recommended in the diagnosis of CAT.

For suspected DVT the gold standard investigation is Doppler ultrasonography which is non-invasive and easily tolerated. Pulmonary emboli are best diagnosed by computer tomography pulmonary arteriography (CTPA). It is important to correlate the clot burden with the clinical symptoms; a small isolated subsegmental PE is unlikely to account for someone's breathlessness whilst a saddle PE with evidence of right heart strain will.

Communication Issues at Diagnosis

Patients frequently report being given little information about VTE at the time of their CAT diagnosis. They describe a rushed and uninformative process which leaves them consulting the internet for guidance, which inevitably exacerbates their distress.[3] This can be minimized with appropriate communication.

The following information should be covered at the point of diagnosis:

- Explain why they got the clot.

  Cancer makes the blood sticky and further cancer treatments can increase this, especially systemic cancer treatments including in the form of tablets.

- Why it is important to treat.

  CAT is easily treatable by using anticoagulants. If untreated, however, the body may create more abnormal clots or the clot already found may get bigger. As well as causing unpleasant symptoms, it can be very dangerous. It may also lead to cancer treatments being withheld or stopped altogether.

- How long it takes for symptoms to improve.

  Most people notice an improvement in symptoms shortly after starting anticoagulants. Anticoagulants work by preventing the formation of further abnormal clots, allowing the body's own fibrinolytic system healing to break down and then absorb the clot. This may take up to three months for symptoms to fully resolve.

- How long they will be anticoagulated for.

  The guidelines recommend 3–6 months anticoagulation. However, if at 6 months there are still signs of active cancer or they are still taking anticancer medicines, it might be necessary to continue anticoagulation longer.

Challenges of Anticoagulation in Cancer Patients

Treatment of VTE in the general population is relatively straight forward. Patients receive 3–6 months of anticoagulation, usually with an oral agent. Since the original precipitant of the thrombus is usually transient e.g., surgery, acute inflammatory illness, immobility, etc., anticoagulation is rarely required beyond this point.

Historically, warfarin was the mainstay of anticoagulation for over 60 years. This has now been superseded by the direct acting oral anticoagulants rivaroxaban, apixaban, edoxaban, and dabigatran (DOACs, also known as non-vitamin K oral anticoagulants by some specialties).

DOACs have several advantages over warfarin, namely:

- Greater safety and efficacy profile.
- They do not require monitoring.

- One dose is recommended for almost all patients.
- Fewer drug interactions.

Anticoagulation in the cancer setting is less straightforward. The rate of VTE recurrence on anticoagulation is high in those with cancer because thrombogenicity is rarely an isolated episode. Risks will vary over time depending on the use of anticancer therapies, disease status, and concurrent illness. Additionally, the risk of bleeding will vary over time particularly when patients are thrombocytopenic due to treatments or marrow infiltration.

Anticoagulation of cancer patients poses risks.[5] These include:

- Increased VTE recurrence compared with non-cancer patients.
- Increased bleeding risk compared non-cancer patients.
- Ongoing and varying risk of VTE.
- Receiving ongoing cancer treatments which may increase risk of VTE, bleeding, and drug–drug interactions.

Initial Treatment of CAT (First 3–6 Months)

The strongest data for the first 3–6 months of treatment of CAT lie with the low molecular weight heparins (LMWH) dalteparin, tinzaparin, and enoxaparin.[6,7]

Despite requiring a daily injection, the main advantages of the LMWHs are:

- Dose is based on patient weight.
- Dose can be adjusted.
- Fewer drug interactions.
- Easy to stop prior to invasive procedures.
- Not affected by vomiting or poor gut absorption.

More recently studies have suggested that apixaban, edoxaban, and rivaroxaban are as effective as LMWH in treating CAT, although some studies have used composite outcomes of recurrent VTE and bleeding rather than recurrent VTE alone.[8] When focussing on recurrent VTE and bleeding separately, DOACs appear slightly better at preventing recurrent DVTs and PEs but this comes at the expense of safety, with bleeding events being more common. The greatest bleeding risk is in patients with gastrointestinal cancers (particularly oesophageal and gastro-oesophageal) and urothelial tumours where the primary tumour remains in situ.[9] In addition, caution should be observed at all times for potential drug–drug interactions particularly strong inducers or inhibitors of cytochrome 3A4 (CYP3A4) and P-glycoprotein (P-Gp).

Another factor associated with increased bleeding is concomitant use of NSAIDs. A recent meta-analysis of 27 papers has recently reported.[10] This paper identifies a significant increase in overall bleeding when comparing NSAIDs used with DOACS vs. DOACs alone (OR = 1.54 95% CI, 1.33 to 1.80; P < 0.00001). There was also significantly increased upper GI bleeding (OR = 2.18; 95% CI, 1.02 to 4.69; P = 0.05). However, no significant increase in major bleeding was observed (OR = 1.42; 95% CI, 0.84 to 2.40; P = 0.19).

When interpreting these data, be mindful that the results were from studies in the non-cancer population anticoagulated for atrial fibrillation or VTE. The increased risk of bleeding in the malignant state is well established and it would be wrong to be falsely reassured by the inconclusive outcomes regarding major bleeds, since these are likely to be greater in patients with cancer.

Deciding upon the most appropriate anticoagulant for treatment of CAT should consider the following factors and be re-assessed throughout the cancer journey.

- Risk of bleeding
- Tumour site
- Suitability of oral medications/absorption
- Drug–drug interactions, especially strong inhibitors or inducers of CYP-3A4 and P-glycoprotein
- Patient preference and values regarding choice of drug

A suggested algorithm for deciding whether to use LMWH or DOAC is illustrated in Figure 3C.1.[11]

As a general rule, and if in doubt, the safest option is to use LWMH. However, the need to administer subcutaneously may be challenging for some patients and compliance is enhanced by good communication explaining the importance of the medicine and how to use it. See Box 3C.1.

BOX 3C.1   TOP TIPS FOR IMPROVING COMPLIANCE WITH SUBCUTANEOUS LMWH

- Reinforce the importance of treating the clot with anticoagulation.
- Explain that if it were possible to use a tablet, you would have done so but this would not be safe/effective in their case because…
- Emphasize that they should NOT expel the air bubble from the LMWH syringe; it is there to minimize bruising.
- Explain that whilst the information leaflets suggest they inject a few cm below the navel (belly button) it is okay for them to inject anywhere they can pinch fat on the abdomen.
- Explain that small bruises are quite normal and often they will heal, as scar tissue leading to subcutaneous lumps is also normal. (Unwarned of this, patients often worry they have cancer deposits under the skin.)
- Do not inject into a lump; it will hurt.
- Rotate injection sites allowing for sore areas to heal.
- Finally, ensure that the patient knows how to get their next prescription of LMWH and that the nominated prescriber has agreed to do this.

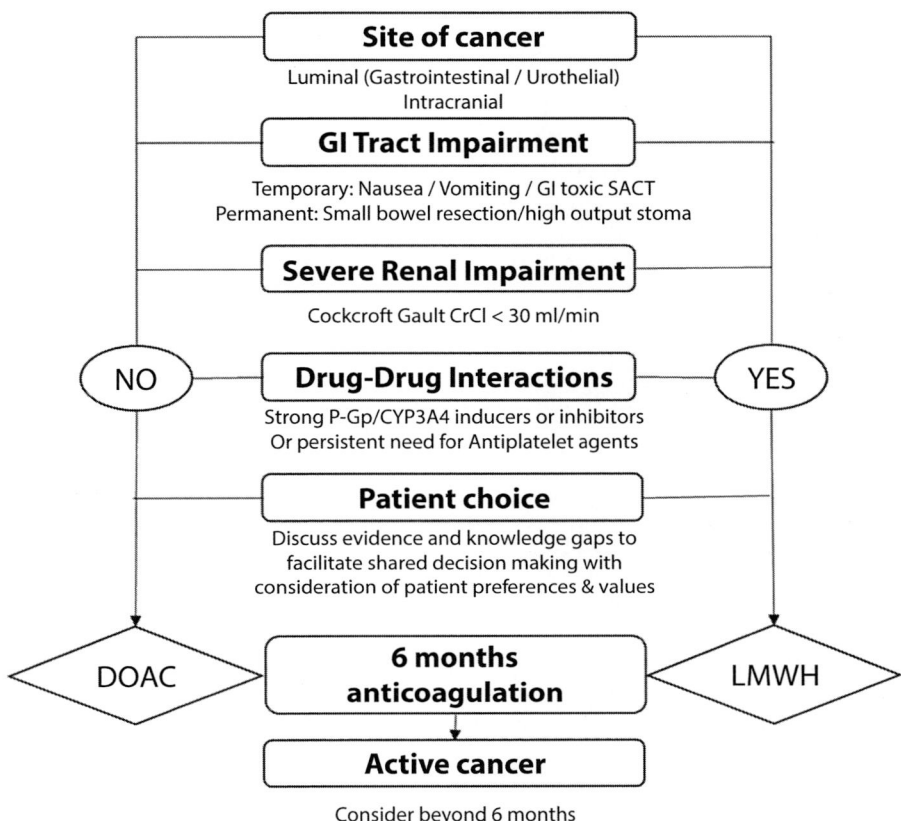

FIGURE 3C.1
Algorithm for choosing between low molecular weight heparin (LMWH) and direct-acting oral anticoagulant (DCAC) for cancer-associated VTE.[12]

Continuing Anticoagulation beyond 6 Months

In patients with ongoing active cancer and/or continuing to receive SACT, it would seem logical to continue anticoagulation since the risk factors for VTE remain. Reputable clinical guidelines recommend the consideration of indefinite anticoagulation in such patients subject to the following considerations:[6,7,13]

- Risk of recurrent thrombosis
- Risk of bleeding
- Patient preferences and values

The choice of which drug to use in the longer term largely depends on patient preference. From clinical experience, only a small number of patients would opt for a LMWH if an oral agent is available. Currently a primary prophylactic dose of DOAC is considered sufficient for long-term secondary prevention although clinical studies are currently underway to identify whether a higher dose of anticoagulant is required and safe.

Incidental Pulmonary Emboli

An incidental pulmonary embolus (PE) is one which has been diagnosed radiologically during imaging undertaken for a different purpose. Due to the increased sensitivity of today's CT scans, they are more commonly being picked up at the point of staging a newly diagnosed cancer and subsequently on follow-up scans to assess disease response to treatment. Sometimes these are called 'asymptomatic PE', although this term is neither useful nor accurate. Close questioning of patients may reveal symptoms associated with PE which have either been considered too mild to mention or attributed to something else.

Even though the symptom burden may be less compared to people presenting with symptomatic PE, the data suggest that those not anticoagulated for incidental PE have poorer survival figures than those who receive anticoagulation.[14]

Communication Issues: Incidental PE[15]

Many patients describe learning about their incidental PEs as "more traumatic than that of being told they had cancer". To understand this in context, we are talking about a patient who has recently been told they have a malignancy (usually by someone who has been on a communication course and hopefully gives the news sensitively).

Incidental PEs, however, are usually identified by the reporting radiologist long after the patient has left the department and returned home. Patients report receiving a telephone call, most likely from someone they haven't met before, to be informed they have found a clot on the lung and need to return to the hospital. To make it worse, this may occur outside office hours and the patient is advised to present to the emergency unit.

Any prevarication by the patient results in being informed: "You must attend immediately. If you don't come in now, you could die." Having already faced their own mortality when diagnosed with cancer, they are once again (and very soon after) informed of another unexpected threat to life. This time the news is given over the phone in an unsatisfactory way without the usual support structures afforded people at their cancer diagnosis.

To make things worse, those who are required to attend the emergency unit of medical admissions often report waiting for hours to be seen (because they look well and are not prioritized) despite attending as a matter of "life and death" urgency. When finally seen, they receive their anticoagulant and are sent home with little information regarding follow-up.

Based on these experiences, it makes sense to develop local pathways for the management of incidental VTE along with appropriate information and follow-up instructions.

Catheter-Related Thrombosis (CRT)

Although previously a relatively common complication, rates of CRT have fallen over the past decade to between 4 and 8%. This is largely due to improvements in insertion techniques, more attention to the site of tip placement, less thrombogenic catheter material, and better line care.

A diagnosis of confirmed CRT does not routinely require line removal. If the catheter is still required for treatment, in the correct position and functioning, removal is not required. Patients should be anticoagulated, preferably with a LMWH as none of the landmark DOAC studies included CRT in the inclusion criteria.

Consensus guidelines recommend a minimum of 3 months' anticoagulation.[7,16] Beyond 3 months, if the catheter remains in situ and/or the patient continues to receive SACT, anticoagulant should continue until provoking risk factors no longer remain.

Intracerebral Tumours

Patients with primary or metastatic brain tumours are at increased risk of VTE with primary gliomas receiving SACT being one of the most thrombogenic malignant conditions. Whilst bleeding on anticoagulation is always a concern, an intratumoural bleed in this situation may be catastrophic. There are a plethora of studies pertaining to the risk of intracranial haemorrhage (ICH) in anticoagulated patients with primary and secondary brain tumours.[16,17]

Thrombocytopenia

Thrombocytopenia is usually due to the cancer or treatment. It is associated with an increased risk of bleeding, especially with anticoagulation. Low platelets do not result in a lower rate of VTE. Anticoagulation should therefore consider the balance of harm from the VTE against the risk of bleeding. If anticoagulation is to be considered, LMWH should be used rather than DOAC. Suggested management of thrombocytopenia in the acute stage of VTE is summarized in Table 3C.1.

Bleeding

Minor bleeding is not uncommon during anticoagulation and most episodes resolve quickly. Recurrent and persistent bleeding should trigger re-evaluation of the need for ongoing anticoagulation or dose modification.

Serious bleeding on anticoagulation occurs in 7% of patients with CAT and is increased in cancers such as glioblastoma, intraluminal gastrointestinal, lung, and bladder cancer. The risk is also greater in metastatic disease, particularly those with highly vascular metastases such as melanoma, renal, thyroid, and testicular cancer. Factors associated with higher risk of significant bleeding are as follows:

- Metastatic disease
- Thrombocytopenia (e.g., chemotherapy, bone marrow failure)

TABLE 3C.1

Management of Thrombocytopenia in Acute VTE (Less than 4 Weeks); Management Should Be Undertaken in Consultation with Haematologist

Platelet Count	High Risk of Thrombosis Recurrence	Low Risk of Thrombosis Recurrence
$>50 \times 10^9/L$	Continue full-dose anticoagulation	Continue full-dose anticoagulation
$25-50 \times 10^9/L$	Consider platelet transfusion to keep the count above $50 \times 10^9/L$ whilst continuing full-dose anticoagulation If not possible consider reducing to intermediate dose	Consider temporarily reducing to prophylactic or intermediate dose
$10-25 \times 10^9/L$	Consider platelet transfusion to keep the count above $25 \times 10^9/L$ Consider temporarily reducing anticoagulation to prophylactic or intermediate dose	Consider temporarily discontinuing anticoagulation Follow normal triggers for platelet transfusion
$<10 \times 10^9/L$	Temporarily discontinue anticoagulation Follow normal triggers for platelet transfusion	Temporarily discontinue anticoagulation Follow normal triggers for platelet transfusion

- Concomitant use with other medicines e.g., NSAIDs, SSRIs
- Poor nutritional status (hypoalbuminemia)
- Recent major bleeding
- Renal dysfunction (creatinine clearance of <30 mL min^{-1})
- Hepatic failure
- Low body weight (<60 kg)

It is important to identify the cause and appropriately manage the bleeding. This will include evaluating whether the patient is over anticoagulated due to drug–drug interactions, reduction in body weight, or drug accumulation due to hepatic or renal impairment. Anticoagulation should be withheld in patients with active, major bleeding, e.g., not amenable to intervention, in a critical site, or life-threatening. In those who are also at high risk of recurrent VTE (e.g., acute or subacute CAT), insertion of a temporary IVC filter may be considered. Once the bleeding has resolved, anticoagulation can be recommenced and the IVC filter removed.[18]

Recurrent VTE on Anticoagulation

Despite the best efforts of us to manage VTE with anticoagulants, a proportion will either fail to respond to anticoagulation or develop further clots whilst fully anticoagulated. Wherever possible, a cause for the recurrent VTE should be considered. Compliance should be checked to identify any interruptions of anticoagulation and a careful history taken to ascertain whether any change in medicines have raised the thrombotic risk.

Heparin-Induced Thrombocytopenia: The Diagnosis Not to Miss

For patients receiving LMWH, a new thrombus in the presence of a drop in platelet count should always raise a suspicion of heparin-induced thrombocytopenia (HIT). The probability of this can be evaluated using the "4Ts" (Table 3C.2) which will be needed to support a request for the diagnostic blood test for antibodies against heparin-PF4.

Recurrent VTE is reported for all anticoagulants in patients with CAT and is as follows:

- 10–17% of those treated with vitamin K antagonist (VKA)
- 6–11% of patients treated with LMWH
- 4–8% of patients treated with DOACs

Is the best way to reduce recurrent VTE to prescribe DOACs every time? Recent research might suggest so, but it is important to recognize that the studies evaluating DOACs were conducted in an arguably healthier patient population with fewer thrombotic risk factors. As such the higher VTE rates in LMWH studies reflected a population with a higher number of patients with metastatic disease and/or receiving SACT.

There are limited data on how to manage recurrent VTE, but the majority of experience lies with the LMWH, where there is the ability to alter drug dosage and availability of anti-Xa level monitoring.[18]

- For patients who develop recurrent VTE whilst taking warfarin, they should be converted to a treatment dose of LMWH according to body weight.
- For those who develop recurrent VTE on LMWH one should first check they have been prescribed the correct dose per body weight as some patients will put on weight during or after cancer treatment, particularly with steroid usage.

TABLE 3C.2

Risk Assessment for Probability of Heparin-Induced Thrombocytopenia (HIT)

Element	The 4T Score for Heparin-Induced Thrombocytopenia	Points
Thrombocytopenia	Fall in platelet count is >50% of the previous value, AND the	2
	lowest count (nadir) is $20–100 \times 10^9$/L	1
	Fall is 30–50% or the nadir is $10–19 \times 10^9$/L	0
	Fall is less than 30% or the nadir is $<10 \times 10^9$/L	
Timing	Fall is after day 10	1
	Exposure to heparin within the last 30 days and then a drop	2
	in platelet count within a day of re-exposure	1
	Previous exposure to heparin 30–100 days ago	0
	Fall is early but there has been no previous heparin exposure	
Thrombosis	New proven thrombosis, skin necrosis, or systemic reaction	2
	Progressive or recurrent thrombosis, silent thrombosis, or red	1
	skin lesions	0
	No symptoms	
Alternative cause possible	No other cause	2
	Possible alternative cause	1
	Definite alternative cause	0

Note: A score of 0–3: HIT is unlikely; 4–5 indicates intermediate probability; 6–8 highly likely.

In patients receiving the correct dose of once-daily LMWH, there are two potential approaches:[17]

1) *Increase LMWH dose by 20–25%*

Two retrospective cohort studies have reported the use of supratherapeutic LWMH to treat recurrent VTE. They recommended empirically increasing the dose by 20–25% and monitoring for symptom improvement. The authors did not use anti-Xa monitoring although this has gained increased popularity in clinical practice.

2) *Change to twice-daily dosing*

The rationale behind this lies with the half-life of LMWHs being approximately 5 hours which means that most patients will have subtherapeutic levels for a significant amount of any given 24-hour period – although whilst making intuitive sense, this method has never been evaluated.

Role of Anti-Xa Level Monitoring

For patients receiving LMWH, anti-Xa levels taken 4 hours after injection may give an indication of drug activity. However, since dosing is given according to body weight, routine anti-Xa monitoring is not recommended.

In clinical practice, anti-Xa levels are helpful in patients with renal failure to establish whether there is drug accumulation.

Anti-Xa levels are also helpful in cases of anticoagulation failure to identify if levels are subtherapeutic or to ensure levels are not dangerously high when using supratherapeutic or BD dosing. Recommended levels vary according to publications but suggested therapeutic anti-Xa levels for low-molecular-weight heparins are:

- 0.5–1.2 U/mL for twice-daily LMWH
- 1.0–1.6 U/mL for once-daily LMWH

Top Tip

Anti-Xa has a half-life of 4 hours. This means that bloods taken in the community are likely to report inaccurately low levels due to the breakdown of anti-Xa prior to arriving at the laboratory. It is therefore advisable to bring patients into hospital to have bloods taken and have them delivered immediately to the laboratory.

Inferior Vena Cava Filters

Inferior vena cava (IVC) filters are a controversial topic in the management of cancer-associated thrombosis. Clinical guidelines are very conservative in recommending their use in the cancer setting, suggesting their use be considered on a case-by-case basis in patients with acute DVT (or PE with evidence of further DVT).[6,7,13,18] This is because of the high risk of complications (see Box 3C.2).

BOX 3C.2 COMPLICATIONS OF IVC FILTER

- **Thrombosis**
  - o 40% incidence of new DVT
  - o Up to 50% will result in caval thrombosis
- **IVC perforation**
  - o Perforation of IVC by filter struts usually incidental
  - o Reported in 50–95%
- **Filter fracture**
  - o 16% reported in one study
- **Pulmonary embolism**
  - o PE reported in up to 5.6%
  - o Fatal PE reported in 3.7% in one study
- **Filter migration**
  - o To another part of the IVC
  - o To the heart
  - o To the pulmonary outflow tract
- **Device infection**
  - o Bacteremia is a contraindication to insertion

The primary purpose of an IVC filter is to prevent fatal pulmonary emboli, although they will not prevent small pulmonary emboli, and neither will they in any way help symptoms of DVT. Furthermore, left in the long term, they can act as a surface for new clot formation, both distal and proximal to their point of placement.

As stated before, current guidelines do not recommend the routine use of IVC filters in patients with cancer and suggest consideration on an individual case-by-case basis. However, they suggest consideration of a temporary (retrievable) IVC filter in patients with acute VTE when interruption in anticoagulation is required during the 4–6 weeks of anti-coagulation (when the clot is at its most unstable and risk of embolizing).

For example: A newly diagnosed cancer patient is found to have pulmonary emboli on a staging scan, and requires surgery. The safest option would be to anticoagulate for 6 weeks, withhold during surgery, and restart again after. If not possible to wait that long, suggest a Doppler ultrasound of both legs to see what DVT was present.

If this is considered, it is imperative that arrangements for retrieval of the filter are considered at the time of insertion. This should ideally be done within 3 months before the filter struts endothelialize, making removal far more challenging and at greater risk of complication.

End of Life

The risk of thrombosis increases with disease progression. Post-mortem studies have shown PE present in 50% of cancer patients. Does this represent an agonal process rather than a terminal event?

Current practice suggests over 50% of anticoagulated cancer patients remain anticoagulated at the time of death. As death approaches, the decision of when to stop anticoagulation (if at all) is a challenging one, due to the high rate of recurrent VTE.[19]

At the end of life, where symptom control is the primary aim, the prevention of death or long-term complications from VTE as clinical aims are no longer relevant. Likewise, patients who have been anticoagulated for longer than 6 months and patients who have been anticoagulated for incidental VTE are unlikely to develop symptomatic VTE in the last weeks of life. Arguably even where VTE symptoms occur at the end of life, they could be managed using end of life medicines such as opioids and benzodiazepines.

In summary, it makes sense to discontinue anticoagulants near the end of life so long as symptom control measures have been put in place. Prior to this, any bleeding episode should be considered a prompt to consider deprescribing of anticoagulants sooner rather than later.

Thromboprophylaxis

The prevention of hospital-associated VTE has been the subject of considerable interest and activity due to the high rate of avoidable harm identified through this phenomenon.

All hospitals should have a thromboprophylaxis policy which should include a risk assessment to identify those most likely to develop VTE. It should also include an evaluation of whether the patient who would be at risk of harm from either pharmacological thromboprophylaxis i.e., low-dose anticoagulants or mechanical thromboprophylaxis i.e., antiembolism stockings or intermittent pneumatic compression. In principle, the presence of cancer should be considered a significant enough risk factor to warrant thromboprophylaxis unless contraindications have been identified (Table 3C.3).

TABLE 3C.3

Contraindications to Thromboprophylaxis

Pharmacological e.g., LMWH
- Coagulopathy INR > 2.0
- Platelet count $<75 \times 10^9$/L
- Active bleeding
- Ischemic or haemorrhagic stroke – discuss with neurology/stroke team
- Traumatic brain injury <72 hr – discuss with neurosurgical team

Use with caution in
- Patients with a recent (within 3 months) history of GI bleeding
- Patients with renal failure as LMWH may accumulate

Mechanical e.g., Anti-Embolism Stockings
- Severe arteriosclerosis or other ischemic vascular diseases
- Severe congestive cardiac failure or any condition where an increase of fluid to the heart may be detrimental
- Known or suspected **acute** DVT, thrombophlebitis, or pulmonary embolism
- Local skin condition likely to be disturbed by stocking e.g. gangrene, a recent skin untreated infected wound

---

Note: LMWH = low molecular weight heparin; DVT = deep vein thrombosis; INR = international normalized ratio hospital inpatients – medical.

No cancer-specific randomized control trials of pharmacological thromboprophylaxis in non-surgical hospitalized inpatients have been published. However, numerous prospective studies have demonstrated an increased risk of VTE in patients hospitalized with an acute medical illness and that pharmacological thromboprophylaxis reduces the risk by approximately 50%.[20]

Subgroup analyses of these studies confirm a higher risk of VTE amongst those with cancer with a similar benefit from pharmacological thromboprophylaxis. Interestingly, pooled data to evaluate the utility of prolonged thromboprophylaxis of medical patients post-discharge identified an increased bleeding risk and it is therefore not recommended.

Hospital Inpatients – Surgical

Cancer patients undergoing surgery are at a higher risk of VTE than those without cancer. Pharmacological thromboprophylaxis with parenteral anticoagulation in cancer patients undergoing surgery is associated with a reduction in post-operative VTE. Extended LMWH thromboprophylaxis studies following abdominal and pelvic surgery demonstrate a reduction in VTE risk by up to 50% compared to less than two weeks' duration, without a significant increase in the risk of major or clinically relevant bleeding.

Whilst the data are not as strong regarding the use of DOACs in the prevention of post-operative VTE in surgical cancer patients, three RCTs (one using apixaban 2.5 mg bd and two using rivaroxaban 10 mg od) have identified them as an acceptable alternative to LMWH[6]

Practice Points: Hospital Thromboprophylaxis

Unless Contraindicated

- Patients with active or recent cancer admitted to hospital with an acute medical illness should receive pharmacological thromboprophylaxis throughout their admission.
- Patients with cancer admitted to hospital for non-minor surgery should receive pharmacological thromboprophylaxis throughout their admission.
- Thromboprophylaxis should be extended to 28 days post-operatively for high-risk surgical patients, such as those requiring surgery for the management of abdominal or pelvic cancer with low molecular weight heparin, or with prophylactic dose rivaroxaban or apixaban after an initial period of LMWH.

Ambulant Cancer Patients Receiving Systemic Anticancer Therapies

Thrombosis is the commonest cause of death during chemotherapy, second only to cancer progression. Mortality and long-term morbidity may be lessened by early diagnosis and treatment yet patient awareness of the signs and symptoms of VTE is very low and not all services have a dedicated VTE pathway to ensure timely management.

Research has shown that patient education about the risks of VTE and what to look out for can reduce the time to presentation, thereby improving outcomes. However, VTE is rarely prioritized during patient chemotherapy education, unlike febrile neutropenia which is managed admirably.

Over 50% of cancer-associated thromboses are diagnosed in the first 3 months of the cancer diagnosis. This is, in part, due to a higher pick-up rate of incidental pulmonary emboli when undertaking a staging CT scan but predominantly due to the use of systemic anticancer therapies (SACT) early in the cancer journey. The numbers needed to treat the general cancer population to prevent one SACT-associated VTE are too high, especially when viewed from an economic perspective. However, with a knowledge that some cancers are particularly prothrombotic, as are particular chemotherapy agents, it makes sense to target patients known to be at particular risk of VTE during treatment.

Multiple Myeloma

Myeloma is associated with an up to 20-fold increased risk of VTE when compared to controls. The risk is increased with corticosteroids and immunomodulatory drugs such as thalidomide, lenalidomide, and pomalidomide. The International Myeloma Working Group (IMWG) recommends patients are risk assessed and receive LMWH prophylaxis for those who are high risk and aspirin for lower risk patients. Several VTE risk scores have been developed including IMPEDE VTE and SAVED (Tables 3C.4 and 3C.5). Whilst these risk assessment scores are derived from clinical data, the recommendations of aspirin and LMWH have not yet been confirmed through prospective randomized control studies.

Pancreatic Cancer

Patients with pancreatic cancer have an extremely high risk of VTE which is further increased by SACT. Two RCTs have focussed on this tumour type using high-dose LMWH

TABLE 3C.4

IMPEDE VTE Myeloma Score

Predictor	Acronym	Score
Immunomodulatory drug	I	+4
Body mass index $\geq$ 25 kg/m^2	M	+1
Pelvic, hip, or femur fracture	P	+4
Erythropoiesis-stimulating agent	E	+1
Doxorubicin	D	+3
Dexamethasone	D	+4
High dose (>160 mg/month)		+2
Standard dose ($\leq$ 160mg/month)		
Ethnicity/ race = Asian Pacific Islander	E	−3
History of venous thromboembolism before multiple myeloma	V	+5
Tunnelled line/central venous catheter	T	+2
Existing thromboprophylaxis: Therapeutic LMWH or warfarin	E	−4
Existing thromboprophylaxis: Prophylactic LMWH or aspirin	E	−3

TABLE 3C.5

SAVED Myeloma Risk Assessment

Predictor	Acronym	Score
Surgery (within 90 days)	S	+2
Asian race	A	−3
History of VTE	V	+3
Eighty (age >80 years)	E	+1
Dexamethasone	D	+2
High dose (>160 mg/cycle)		+1
Standard dose (120–160 mg/cycle)		

TABLE 3C.6

Khorana Risk Assessment Tool

Characteristic	Points
Cancer site: Very high-risk (stomach, pancreas)	+2
Cancer site: High risk (lung, lymphoma, gynaecological, bladder, testicular)	+1
Pre-chemo platelets ≥350 × 10^9/L	+1
Hb <100 g/L or use of erythrocyte stimulating agent	+1
Pre-chemo WCC >11 × 10^9/L	+1
BMI ≥35 kg/m^2	+1

Note: 0 = low; 1–2 = intermediate; ≥3 = high risk (from ref 23 with permission).

schedules during their first line chemotherapy. One study used full therapeutic dose dalteparin for 12 weeks and the other enoxaparin (1 mg/kg).[21,22] Both regimes observed over 80% reduction in VTE compared to their respective control arms with no increase in bleeding complications. Patients with pancreatic cancer were also included in the studies of targeted DOAC thromboprophylaxis is those identified at high risk of VTE (Khorana score ≥2). Clinical guidelines therefore suggest thromboprophylaxis for ambulant pancreatic cancer patients embarking on chemotherapy.

Other Cancers

Primary prophylaxis with LMWH has been shown to reduce VTE rates by 50% in numerous studies but the high heterogeneity of participants meant that it was difficult to recommend prophylaxis for all ambulant cancer patients receiving SACT. Identification of those at highest risk would allow them to be targeted with thromboprophylaxis. Many cancer-specific VTE risk assessment scores have been developed. The most used and evaluated is the Khorana score[23] (Table 3C.6) which predicts thrombosis risk based on cancer type, routine bloods, and body mass index.

Practice Points: Thromboprophylaxis in Ambulant Cancer Patients Receiving SACT

In the absence of contraindications, in patients commencing SACT:

- Myeloma patients deemed high risk by a myeloma-specific risk assessment score should be offered pharmacological thromboprophylaxis.
- Pancreatic cancer patients should be offered pharmacological thromboprophylaxis with an anticoagulant in line with the dosage used in clinical trials.
- Ambulatory cancer patients identified as high risk on a validated VTE score who are embarking on SACT may be considered for pharmacological thrombopropylaxis.

Cancer-associated thrombosis will continue to be a challenge for clinicians involved in supportive oncology and the number of cases will increase. This is because patients are living longer with metastatic disease and receiving more systemic anticancer therapies.

The heterogeneity of the cancer patient according to primary, stage, and treatment modalities is considerable and a "one size fits all" approach to CAT treatment or prevention is becoming increasingly outdated.

As a time where cancer management is so personalized that cancer treatment choices are guided by genetic mutations or protein expression, it should not be unreasonable to adopt a more individualized approach to CAT, and possible advances in AI technology may play a pivotal part in identifying risk and stratifying patients for optimum care in the future.

Furthermore, as CAT management becomes more complex, the importance of a multi-professional approach involving close liaison with haematology services cannot be over-emphasized.

References

1. Kumar DR et al. Virchow's contribution to the understanding of thrombosis and cellular biology. *Clin Med Res.* 2010;8(3–4):168–72.
2. Noble S, Pasi J. Epidemiology and pathophysiology of cancer-associated thrombosis. *Br J Cancer.* 2010;102(Suppl 1):S2–9.
3. Noble S et al. Patients' experiences of living with cancer-associated thrombosis: the PELICAN study. *Patient Prefer Adherence.* 2015;9:337–45.
4. Kelly J, Hunt BJ. Role of D-dimers in diagnosis of venous thromboembolism. *Lancet.* 2002;359(9305):456–8.
5. Khorana AA et al. Cancer-associated venous thromboembolism. *Nat Rev Dis Primers.* 2022;8(1):11.
6. Lyman GH et al. American Society of Hematology 2021 guidelines for management of venous thromboembolism: prevention and treatment in patients with cancer. *Blood Adv.* 2021;5(4):927–74.
7. Falanga A et al. Venous thromboembolism in cancer patients: ESMO clinical practice guideline. *Ann Oncol.* 2023;34(5):452–67.

8. Khorana AA et al. Role of direct oral anticoagulants in the treatment of cancer-associated venous thromboembolism: guidance from the SSC of the ISTH. *J Thromb Haemost*. 2018;16(9):1891–4.

9. Raskob GE et al. Edoxaban for the treatment of cancer-associated venous thromboembolism. *N Engl J Med*. 2018;378(7):615–24.

10. Zheng Y et al. Co-administered oral anticoagulants with nonsteroidal anti-inflammatory drugs and the risk of bleeding: A systematic review and meta-analysis. *Thromb Res*. 2023;232:15–26.

11. Carrier M et al. Treatment algorithm in cancer-associated thrombosis: updated Canadian expert consensus. *Curr Oncol*. 2021;28(6):5434–51.

12. Alikhan R et al. Cancer-associated venous thrombosis in adults (second edition): A British society for haematology guideline. *Br J Haematol*. 2024;205(1):71–87.

13. Khorana AA et al. Guidance for the prevention and treatment of cancer-associated venous thromboembolism. *J Thromb Thrombolysis*. 2016;41(1):81–91.

14. Liebman HA, O'Connell C. Incidental venous thromboembolic events in cancer patients: what we know in 2016. *Thromb Res*. 2016;140 (Suppl 1):S18–20.

15. Noble S et al. Patient experience of living with cancer-associated thrombosis in Canada (PELICANADA). *Res Pract Thromb Haemost*. 2020;4(1):154–60.

16. Iyengar V et al. Comparison of direct oral anticoagulants versus low-molecular-weight heparin in primary and metastatic brain cancers: a meta-analysis and systematic review. *J Thromb Haemost*. 2024;22(2):423–9.

17. Zwicker J. Prevention and treatment of venous thromboembolism in primary and metastatic brain cancer. *Clin Adv Hematol Oncol*. 2022;20(10):594–6.

18. Carrier M et al. Management of challenging cases of patients with cancer-associated thrombosis including recurrent thrombosis and bleeding: guidance from the SSC of the ISTH. *J Thromb Haemost*. 2013;11(9):1760–5.

19. Noble S et al. Management of venous thromboembolism in far-advanced cancer: current practice. *BMJ Support Palliat Care*. 2022;12(e6):e834–7.

20. NICE. Venous thromboembolism in over 16s: reducing the risk of hospital-acquired deep vein thrombosis or pulmonary embolism. *NICE Guideline [NG89]*, 2018, available at: https://www.nice.org.uk/guidance/ng89.

21. Maraveyas A et al. Gemcitabine versus gemcitabine plus dalteparin thromboprophylaxis in pancreatic cancer. *Eur J Cancer*. 2012;48(9):1283–92.

22. Pelzer U et al. Primary pharmacological prevention of thromboembolic events in ambulatory patients with advanced pancreatic cancer treated with chemotherapy. *Dtsch Med Wochenschr*. 2013;138(41):2084–8.

23. Khorana AA et al. Development and validation of a predictive model for chemotherapy-associated thrombosis. *Blood*. 2008;111(10):4902–7.

Section III

Rehabilitation and Survivorship

4

Survivorship and Late Consequences of Treatment

4A

Survivorship and Personalized Care

Ben Heyworth and James Burtonwood

Introduction

Most health care professionals now recognize that the complex challenges faced by patients living with and beyond cancer may require specialized, person-centred support, both with the management of ongoing consequences of treatment and late effects, and the emotional, psychological, vocational, spiritual, and social impact of disease. Many patients will be seeking to settle into what could be described as a "new normal", where maintaining as good a quality of life as possible following a period of recuperation and rehabilitation is critical.[1]

Survivorship is considered by some to begin from the moment of diagnosis; however using the label 'survivor' as a For some patients this is an affirmative, empowering term, whereas others find it offensive.[2] In the light of this, some professionals are more likely to use the phrase 'living with and beyond cancer'.

'Living with and beyond cancer' includes those individuals who are in remission, treated with curative intent, and essentially disease-free. These people are primarily interested in promoting and sustaining their recovery.

It also refers to those patients who are living with incurable but managed disease, for whom quality of life and living well are important, as well as minimizing and managing any disease or treatment-related symptoms and promoting resilience and emotional wellbeing.

Some professionals also consider individuals who have a life-limiting illness to be part of this group, where maintaining quality of life and emotional resilience is important for a few years before moving into palliative or end of life care setting.

In any case, patients who might be considered "living with and beyond" represent a diverse intersection of individuals with many contrasting needs and concerns.

Optimal patient engagement in follow-up care and potentially through supportive oncology MDTs is essential not only because multiple and complex late consequences of treatment can occur many years after treatment has concluded, but also because the impact

DOI: 10.1201/9781003369912-9

of cancer in the broadest possible sense can often take a long time to resolve. Effective models of care should ensure effective monitoring for disease reoccurrence, the possibility of which is a significant driver for anxiety amongst individuals in follow-up and beyond, as well as adequate signposting to services that can assist with a range of other concerns which may include, but not be limited to, support with financial issues, social care, relationship counselling, sexual health and wellbeing, and employment.

Quality cancer survivorship care should aim to empower people living with and beyond cancer by encouraging patients to be active participants in managing their care. Services should be sustainable and scalable as the number of patients living with and beyond cancer continues to increase and offer value for money to the local health and social care systems.[3]

A systematic approach that combines redesigning follow-up and survivorship clinical pathways, enhanced patient information around the consequences of treatment and wellbeing, and the recording of patient outcome data can significantly improve the ability of professionals to manage the myriad challenges faced by patients 'living with and beyond'.[4]

It is likely that survivorship care will be delivered in multiple care settings and by a range of organizations, perhaps leaning further into primary care and community-based services as the pathway extends further from the end of acute treatment settings. Therefore, the complex issue of managing the operational intersections between acute, tertiary, and primary care services must be addressed by providers: Including sharing the responsibility of care and associated patient data, and recognizing a growing role for voluntary and community-based enterprises (VCSE) within integrated health care systems that can offer bespoke, local interventions that have the potential to significantly improve the level and type of support that is available to individuals near to where they live.

Epidemiology of "Living with and beyond Cancer"

In England, five-year survival rates have improved for most cancers in adults, and the 5-year survival for childhood cancers has seen the highest increase ever recorded, from 76.9% in 2002 to 85.0% in 2019.[5] Richards et al.[6] predict the number of people described as "living with and beyond" cancer will rise to 4 million by 2030. Improvements in mortality data are undoubtably good news for cancer patients, but it is important to note that the picture is not the same across every disease group. Where cancer survival rates are highest, for example in melanoma of the skin, where 5-year survival for both males is 89.9% and females 94.8%, there are likely to be many more individuals living with and beyond. Where cancer survival is lowest, in pancreatic cancer and mesothelioma, where 5-year survival is lowest for mesothelioma in males (6.3%) and pancreatic cancers in females (7.8%), it is unlikely that large numbers of patients would be in the survivorship part of the pathway.[5]

Similarly, cancer survival varies by stage at diagnosis. Five-year survival by stage ranges from 3.2% (stage 4 lung cancer for males) to 101.1% (stage 1 melanoma for females) – and clearly those patients who are diagnosed early are more likely to live with and beyond and are less likely to encounter complex survivorship challenges.[5]

As Sarah Lochlann Jain describes in her 2007 paper "Living in Prognosis: Towards an Elegiac Politics",[7] the epidemiology of survivorship suggests "a sense of order amid the chaos of disease … a thin veneer of certainly while simultaneously hollowing out any tangible meaning", and indeed, there is evidence to suggest that patients arrive at the point where they might be considered "living beyond" cancer with a renewed sense of uncertainty and in some cases foreboding, particularly when treatment has been stopped and innovative new follow-up pathway arrangements reduce the regularity and consistency of support from health care professionals.

Personalized Stratified Follow-up

Follow-up after cancer treatment has traditionally been a standardized affair – regular appointments as a default, at an interval largely determined by a local protocol. For many years, there has been an assumption that regular, planned follow-up improves detection of early or asymptomatic recurrence and thus improves survival. Many contemporary studies paint a different picture. Patients with recurrence after treatment for stage one endometrial cancer, for example, have no difference in survival regardless of whether recurrence is detected during routine planned follow-up or in those re-presenting urgently with symptoms.[8] Similarly, intensive follow-up in colorectal cancer does not improve survival.[9]

As the prevalence of cancer survivorship in the population increases and survival improves, this 'regular follow-up by default' model places an increasingly heavy burden on health care services which need to accommodate ever more patients over longer periods. Thus, the follow-up clinic appointment becomes an increasingly precious commodity, resulting in less time dedicated to patient-centred care or identification of treatment-related complications. Patients may be recalled for appointments they don't need or want which may contribute to the 'time-toxicity' of cancer treatment.[10] Conversely, those in pressing need of review may find themselves waiting longer than necessary. Thus, the original 'one size fits all' approach to follow-up increasingly appears to be 'one size fits none'.

The NHS 2021 long-term plan included ambitions that every person diagnosed with cancer will have access to personalized care. Personalized stratified follow-up (PSFU) has been increasingly adopted as a strategy to deliver this goal. Over and above the stated drive for personalized care, it is hoped that PSFU could allow significant redeployment of outpatient slots thus relieving the pressures on outpatient services. NHS England estimate that per 1000 referrals, over 5 years, PSFU could free up 2850 follow-up clinic appointments for breast, 2750 for colorectal, and 1900 for prostate cancers.[11]

PSFU is an umbrella term for a more nuanced mechanism for meeting the needs of cancer survivors and encompasses a variety of similar patient-centred initiatives. There is wide variation in the terms used to describe the process at a local level. Fundamentally, however, patients receiving PSFU may be allocated to one of two routes, namely:

- Patient initiated follow-up (PIFU) sometimes known as supported self-management.
- Or clinician led follow-up (CLFU) also known as personalized timed follow-up or scheduled follow-up.

Undoubtably, supportive oncology MDTs will encounter patients stratified into both models of follow-up, or indeed find themselves taking clinical responsibility for the management of either or both follow-up pathways.

There is significant heterogeneity in the approaches taken to implement PSFU (as evidenced by the wide variation in nomenclature). Outcome data is largely collated at a local level so the wider picture of the adoption and effectiveness of PIFU is still emerging.

Nevertheless, PIFU appears to provide a good foundation for empowering patients and providing personalized care, although the effectiveness of PIFU as a safe and effective follow-up strategy is partly dependent on the cancer in question; the pattern and risk of recurrence need to be well-defined and understood. Careful administration is required to avoid "losing" patients to follow-up. There may also be a risk of patients not reporting symptoms of concern in a timely fashion.[12]

Care must be taken to ensure that PIFU is appropriate so that those with more complex needs are adequately cared for. For example, patients with learning disabilities may be less able to identify symptoms of concern and those with restricted autonomy (such as prisoners) may be less enabled to access timely review. An intersectional, individualized approach is required to avoid PIFU worsening health inequalities.

Many patients on a CLFU pathway value the psychological safety of regular, scheduled contact with a health care professional. Regular contact may mitigate the fear of recurrence which tends to return between appointments. Components of post-treatment follow-up have been identified which are particularly valued by patients: Effective mechanisms to communicate with the cancer team, effective information sharing, and psychological support.[12]

Supportive oncology teams should also consider a mechanism for patients to move between pathways as clinical need, circumstances, and patient wishes dictate.

Health and Wellbeing Information and Support in a Digital Age

In many parts of the world the social stigma demanding conversations about cancer should be reduced to hushed asides obliquely referring to "The Big C" has significantly reduced and there has been a proliferation of podcasts, websites, TV documentaries, social media, and informal networks. Such prolificacy of information inevitably impacts the psychological and emotional wellbeing of patients referred into supportive oncology particularly those patients who might be on a PIFU protocol.

Whilst many cancer patients want to be kept informed about their illness,[13] patients vary in how much information they want, and this may change. Patients over 70 years of age generally prefer to leave the disclosure of information about disease to their doctor; however results from this very large study suggest that the vast majority of patients with cancer want a great deal of specific information concerning their illness and treatment.[14]

For many people living with and beyond cancer, it is only through access and interpretation of cancer stories supported by accurate cancer information that they can begin to construct and own a personal survivorship narrative that ultimately leads to defining their "new normal" and their expectations of what life will now be like going forward.

Some patients are more likely than others to take the initiative when it comes to researching their disease independently,[15] with some groups (men) more conspicuously less likely to become active participants.[16] Evidence suggests that some 'self-activated' patients turn to the internet to research symptoms, treatments, and therapies, attend online support groups, and use discussion boards.[17]

In the highly networked and information heavy 21st century, where 92% of people report having regular access to a smartphone,[18] what counts as "reliable" cancer information and support has broadened, and instant access via mobile devices has now become the norm, but what passes as 'reliable' can just as easily be someone's opinion, a sales pitch, or a malicious actor. Has rapid access to misleading information online now become a critical patient safety issue?

Should the traditional gatekeepers of clinical information, the multi-disciplinary team, have a role in managing patient access to online cancer information?

A publication from Greenfield et al.[19] interviewed both cancer experts and general practitioners (GPs) on long-term follow-up provision for cancer survivors and suggested that learning more about late effects and checking for cancer recurrence were rated as the most important reasons for follow-up by cancer experts. The study suggested that respondents valued clinical reasons for follow-up more highly than supportive reasons: Arguably, therefore, a debate should be had around to what extent clinicians should be responsible for providing wellbeing and information needs. Perhaps there is a greater role for voluntary and community-based organizations who are perhaps more readily able to adopt an intersectional approach to delivering the right information at the right time, in the right way.

There are also legitimate concerns that a patient can come across seemingly contradictory information online that plays to an existing unconscious bias or perhaps offers a more appealing 'version' of the truth, which is not supported by the clinical team.

More research needs to be undertaken to assess the extent and effectiveness of cancer health and wellbeing information and support delivered to patients on risk stratified pathways.

Vocational Rehabilitation and Stigma

When considering the socio-cultural impact of cancer for people of working age many individuals view a return to employment as a significant milestone in their recovery, a step 'back to normal' that not only reduces the perceived stigma associated with unemployment, but also recognizes the value in altered bodies that are able to reclaim a reasonable level of pre-cancer functionality, and in many instances an uninhibited return to full-time employment.[20]

Lack of advice from clinical teams around successfully managing a return to the workplace has been cited as a barrier to reclaiming employment, but not all clinicians will consider themselves to be sufficiently knowledgeable to offer advice on this topic. Similarly, should patients have good relations with their employer/line manager, this appears to be a major influence on whether a patient successfully returns to employment, in combination with longer lengths of service.[21]

Supportive oncology teams may not always be best placed to directly assist patients who need to have conversations with their employers around workplace stigmas or making reasonable adjustments to get back to work, but all clinicians working with people living with and beyond cancer should be able to signpost patients to agencies where support may be available. This might include hospital-based services, cancer information centres, or voluntary and community sector organizations, some of which may specialize in offering this type of support.

The Role of Primary Care

Although the face of primary care has changed significantly over the years, the focus on preventative medicine, holistic care of patients and families, management of complex co-morbidity, and early diagnosis of malignancy all remain core remits. Primary care can and should play a vital role in caring for people living with and beyond cancer.

Many survivorship issues are closely aligned with the services and benefits primary care offers[22] and these include the promotion of good cardiovascular health, managing the impact of cancer on mental health and wellbeing, being alert for signs of recurrent disease, and help with sexual function.

Similarly, most primary care practices have dedicated specialized teams experienced in adjusting the myriad of new diabetic treatments available and may prove valuable allies for supportive oncology teams treating diabetic patients and other co-morbidities impacted by a cancer diagnosis.

This is particularly vital when we consider that the risk of cardiovascular disease (CVD) is greater in those with cancer even before the modifying impact of cancer treatment effects on this risk. Efforts to reduce baseline cardiovascular risk, both as pre-habilitation measures, but also throughout the life of cancer survivors, is a key area in which primary care teams may help to reduce the excess morbidity and mortality resulting from cancer treatments.

Similarly, primary care teams, experienced in the management of hypertension, are well-placed to monitor, to escalate anti-hypertensive therapy, and crucially to rationalize and de-prescribe therapy if hypertension resolves on treatment cessation. Primary care teams may also have many survivors of childhood cancer amongst their patient populations. These patients, who may have been exposed to anthracycline chemotherapy, may be particularly prone to asymptomatic cardiomyopathy.

Anxiety and depression are common in cancer survivors and the prevalence of these conditions may far exceed that amongst the general population.[23] Cancer survivors may have complex psychological needs which may change over time[24] and there may also be important biological inputs such as the cytokine IL-6-mediated depression sometimes seen in pancreatic cancer or iatrogenic premature menopause. Finally, there also numerous treatment effects to consider such as androgen deprivation therapy, panhypopituitarism in immunotherapy, or direct depressant effects of chemotherapy agents such as paclitaxel or vincristine.[25]

As discussed in Chapter 4B, the last few years has seen a steady increase in specialist late effect clinics yet only about 20% of patients with GI or pelvic late effects will be managed in specialist care.[26] Patients may experience chronic syndromes, indolent symptoms, or late onset of symptoms. Given the expected increase in prevalence of cancer survivors and the associated symptom burden, cancer specialists may need to turn increasingly to shared-care models and provide additional support and education to patients and primary care services alike to meet the need.

In the UK, perhaps one of the greatest impacts which primary care has on population health is the co-ordination and delivery of vaccination programmes. Effective vaccination requires a competent immune system and vaccinations such as pneumococcus, for example, are advised at least two weeks before the beginning of chemotherapy for full seroconversion. In the flurry of clinical activity following a cancer diagnosis, patients may miss this 'window of opportunity'. An important part of survivorship care in general practice should be to ensure vaccination schedules are followed. Similarly, there may be certain cases where immunosuppression is expected to continue after cancer treatments in which case cancer specialists need to have reliable methods of communicating when certain routine live vaccinations, such as attenuated herpes zoster, would be contra-indicated.

Without encouragement and direction, it may be difficult for primary care teams to recognize and conduct proactive case-finding of at-risk patients amongst their population[27] so perhaps key to joint management of CV risk for survivors is clear communication between specialists and primary care.

There is increasing recognition of the importance of chemoprophylaxis in certain cancers. For example, the role of aspirin in prevention of Lynch syndrome is now well-recognized, and selective oestrogen receptor modulators are increasingly used to prevent cancers in patients with genetic pre-disposition to breast cancer. Fundamental to this preventative approach is the recognition of at-risk families by primary care teams. ESC teams may be able to assist this whole-family approach by clear communication of potentially inheritable cancers (such as colorectal or endometrial cancers in Lynch syndrome, or BRCA-related cancers). This can allow primary care to undertake a wider family risk assessment followed by referral to genetic services where appropriate.

Many of the lifestyle modifications discussed above are crucial in reducing the risk of secondary malignancies; primary care may play a vital role in the further modification of risk factors such as alcohol and smoking. Many working in the community are well-placed to be able to signpost and prescribe lifestyle measures and other risk-modifying behavioural treatments such as local exercise classes, smoking cessation services, gym memberships, and diet-modification groups.

Strategic and Service Development in the United Kingdom

A significant national strategy intervention from NHS Improvement and Macmillan Cancer Support in the period 2010–2013 considerably advanced the introduction of new models of care to support patients living with and beyond cancer. The National Cancer Survivorship Initiative (NCSI) built on the Cancer Reform Strategy (DH 2007) and recognized that more needed to be done to support the growing numbers of patients in the Survivorship part of the pathway.

Supported through the National Cancer Survivorship Initiative (2010) and recognizing that the management of the late consequences of treatment was a key clinical challenge, a number of initiatives across the UK, most notably at the Sheffield Teaching Hospital NHS Foundation Trust (led by Prof. Diana Greenfield) and at the Royal Marsden in London (led by Dr Jervais Andreyev), were created to pilot interventions and service improvements, and drive research and education. Dr Andreyev recognized early on that improvements in treatment options for cancer largely bypassed non-oncologists who do not always fully understand the interventions which have been used and that much cancer care is delivered in 'stand-alone' cancer centres where expert supportive care by other specialties is not always available.[26] Prof. Greenfield was instrumental in driving new research and developing successful care models for nurse-led interventions in survivorship care and the management of complex late consequences of treatment.

The introduction of the "Recovery Package" over the last 15 years has made a significant and lasting difference to the support patients received as they moved beyond treatment, as it included requirements for all patients to have holistic assessments and care plans, access to health and wellbeing "events", and improved communication between specialists and primary care – but successful implementation across the NHS was far from universal. By 2022, the Recovery Package had been largely subsumed into the "Personalised Care" framework, which took a less prescriptive but equally holistic approach to managing patients, and in principle is transferable to patients with other long-term conditions. It is becoming more common when speaking about patients living with and beyond cancer to contextualize the topic within the parameters of personalized care; however it remains to be seen if newly designed and implemented PCFU pathways fully embrace the principle of risk stratification as originally articulated in 2010 by NHS Improvement and Macmillan Cancer Support, and deliver both improvements to the quality of care for patients and create the required capacity within the system to accommodate the increasing numbers of patients who could be described as living with and beyond.

References

1. Hewitt M et al. *From Cancer Patient to Cancer Survivor: Lost in Translation: National Research Council.* Washington, DC: National Academies Press; 2005.
2. Berry L et al. Is it time to reconsider the term 'cancer survivor'? *J Psychosoc Oncol* 2019;37(4):413–426.
3. Loonen J et al. Cancer survivorship care: person centered care in a multidisciplinary shared care model. *Int J Integrated Care.* 2018;18(1):4.
4. Maher EJ. Managing the consequences of cancer treatment and the English national cancer survivorship initiative. *Acta Oncol.* 2013;52(2):225–232.
5. NHS Digital. Cancer survival in England, cancers diagnosed 2015 to 2019, followed up to 2020 [internet], 2022. Available at: https://digital.nhs.uk/data-and-information/publications/statistical/cancer-survival-in-england/cancers-diagnosed-2015-to-2019-followed-up-to-2020#.
6. Richards M et al. The national cancer survivorship initiative: new and emerging evidence on the ongoing needs of cancer survivors. *Br J Cancer.* 2011;105(Suppl 1):S1–S4.
7. Jain L. Living in prognosis: toward an elegiac politics. *Representations* 2007;98(1):77–92.
8. Gadducci A. et al. An intensive follow-up does not change survival of patients with clinical stage I endometrial cancer. *Anticancer Res* 2000;20(3B):1977–1984.
9. Jeffery M et al. Follow-up strategies for patients treated for non-metastatic colorectal cancer. *Cochrane Database Syst Rev.* 2019(9).
10. Gupta A et al. The time toxicity of cancer treatment. *J Clin Oncol* 2022;40(15):1611–1615.
11. NHS England and NHS Improvement. Implementing personalised stratified follow up pathways: a handbook for local health and care systems [internet], 2020, available at: https://www.england.nhs.uk/wp-content/uploads/2020/04/cancer-stratified-follow-up-handbook-v1-march-2020.pdf [accessed July 2023].
12. Lewis RA et al. Patients' and healthcare professionals' views of cancer follow-up: systematic review. *Br J General Practice* 2009;59(564):e248–e259.
13. Meredith Cal. Information needs of cancer patients in West Scotland: cross sectional survey of patients' views. *BMJ* 1996;313:724–726.
14. Jenkins V et al. Information needs of patients with cancer: results from a large study in UK cancer centres. *Br J Cancer* 2001;84(1):48–51.
15. Leydon GM et al. Cancer patients' information needs and information seeking behaviour: in depth interview study. *BMJ* 2000;320:909.
16. Moynihan C et al. *Strength in Silence: Men and Cancer,* British Psychosocial Oncology conference, Royal College of Physicians, London, 1999.
17. Falisi AL et al. Social media for breast cancer survivors: a literature review. *J Cancer Survivorship* 2017;11:808.
18. Deloitte, Global Mobile Consumer Trends, second edition [internet], 2022, available at: https://www.deloitte.com/global/en/Industries/tmt/perspectives/gx-global-mobile-consumer-trends.html.

19. Greenfield DM et al. Follow-up care for cancer survivors: the views of clinicians. *Br J Cancer* 2009;101(4):568–574.

20. Kennedy F et al. Returning to work following cancer: a qualitative exploratory study into the expereince of returning to work following cancer. *Eur J Cancer Care,* 2007;16:17–25.

21. Amir Z et al. Cancer survivors' views of work 3 years post diagnosis: a UK perspective. *Eur J Oncol Nursing* 2008;12(3):190–1907.

22. Manthri S et al. Overview of cancer survivorship care for primary care providers. *Cureus* 2020;12(9):e10210.

23. Niedzwiedz CL et al. Depression and anxiety among people living with and beyond cancer: a growing clinical and research priority. *BMC Cancer* 2019;19(1):943.

24. Pascoe SW. Psychosocial care for cancer patients in primary care? Recognition of opportunities for cancer care. *Family Practice* 2004;21(4):437–442.

25. Pitman A et al. Depression and anxiety in patients with cancer. *Br Med J* 2018;361:k1415.

26. Andreyev H et al. Practice guidance on the management of acute and chronic gastrointestinal problems arising as a result of treatment for cancer. *Gut* 2012;61(2):179–192.

27. Bates JE et al. Therapy-related cardiac risk in childhood cancer survivors: an analysis of the childhood cancer survivor study. *J Clin Oncol* 2019;37(13):1090–1101.

4B

Late Consequences of Treatment

Anna Olsson-Brown, Emma Hallam, and Lisa Durrant

Defining Late Effects in Modern Oncology

It is estimated around one in four people with cancer are living with long-term consequences of treatment.[1] Evidence on which problems are the most burdensome remains scarce, although several research studies have been undertaken concluding that there is a need for ongoing support.[2]

> While quality of life in disease-free breast cancer survivors 5 years post-diagnosis was largely comparable to the general population on average, still many survivors suffered from adverse effects. There appears to be a need for ongoing screening and support regarding fatigue, sleep problems, cognitive problems, arthralgia/pain, menopausal/ sexual symptoms, physical performance, and weight problems during and several years following breast cancer therapy.[2]

In another study by Schmidt,[3] more than one-third of disease-free cancer survivors reported specific physical, psychological, cognitive, social, and sexual problems four years after diagnosis. The most common issues reported were loss of physical performance (36.3%), fatigue (35.1%), sexual problems (34.7%), sleep issues (34.1%), arthralgia (33.8%), anxiety (28.0%), neuropathy (25.6%), and memory issues (23.0%).

Other areas of concern included fertility, sexual health and menopause, respiratory and cardiac function, lymphoedema, chronic pain, psychological issues, late toxicities, effects on the bladder and bowel, osteoporosis, and secondary malignancies (particularly for those experiencing their first malignancy in childhood). Significant determinants were identified, including prior chemotherapy, obesity, and cancer type, and patients often rated care satisfaction as poor.

Schmidt et al. highlight the long-term and late effects of treatment that cancer patients experience and support the development of evidence-based, tailored survivorship plans. They also recognize that both the awareness of health care professionals regarding this burden and investment into services to support improvement in the area are required.

In aiming to support patients there have been a variety of late-effect support models and services that have evolved over time. In some private US cancer centres, specialist survivorship nursing roles have been developed; these nurses are central to the management of patients in medium-/long-term recovery and can refer patients into integrated specialist services for appropriate interventions and support. Social workers manage the more holistic elements of a survivorship care plan, and access to complementary therapies and other support is available for most patients – in many ways, a gold standard service.

DOI: 10.1201/9781003369912-10

In the UK, there is no overall transfer of clinical responsibility to a specialist survivorship team; however UK services often include a focus on late effects in specific populations. These include stem cell transplant patients, paediatric, teenage and young adult patients (as discussed in Chapter 6B), patients receiving pelvic radiotherapy, and, increasingly, patients receiving immunotherapy. There are also a number of therapeutic radiographer-led services, many offering management for common radiotherapy-induced late effects. Paediatric patients and specific patient groups benefit from consensus guidelines and long-term follow-up plans, whereas most adults are disadvantaged by a lack of specific guidance and underdeveloped services.[4]

In many cancer centres, there is an increasing recognition of the deleterious cardiac effects of high-intensity treatments. Cardio-oncology services, where cardiologists specialize in the cardiotoxic late effects of treatment, are being rapidly developed.

Managing patients with an ongoing cancer burden is distinct from those that no longer have cancer but are managing the ongoing consequences of treatment; however both groups can and do experience late effects of treatment. This is an evolving area of practice as historically cancer survival whilst receiving palliative treatment was limited – late effects were only recognized in the curative setting. Due to the efficacy, numeracy, and duration of treatment a patient now may experience late effects from one treatment whilst receiving another. This may lead to lack of clarity regarding leadership of care and the management of the different issues.

Late Effects of Radiotherapy

Late effects of radiotherapy are common and include any side-effects resulting from treatment that persist or develop several months or years after treatment has finished. Radiotherapy is a highly effective treatment; however many patients will experience unintended consequences as a result. The number of people affected is rising year on year.

Whilst there are techniques being developed to try and reduce morbidity, such as stereotactic ablative body radiotherapy (SABR) and proton beam therapy, there are still likely to be some late effects from these modalities and a significant lag in understanding the impact of these therapies on the likelihood and severity of potential late effects.

The vast majority of patients continue to receive external beam radiotherapy and a study from the USA suggested that there will be 4.17 million cancer survivors treated with radiotherapy by 2030, many of whom will have had radiotherapy known to be highly related to late effects including breast (40%), prostate (23%), head and neck (5.8%), lymphoma (5.6%), uterine (3.9%), and rectal cancer (3.8%).[5]

Following treatment, many patients will present months (or even decades) later due to radiation-induced fibrosis (RIF). RIF is a progressive fibrotic sclerosis with varying clinical symptoms that stiffens connective tissue and compresses peripheral nerve tracts, contributing to diminished strength and flexibility and loss of function. Often RIF is a debilitating and lifelong progressive disorder resulting in a negative impact on not only function but quality of life.[6]

Referrals for RIF are usually from patients at 6 months and onwards following completion of treatment. Support and advice are offered to help patients to live well with the physical and psychological consequences. It must be noted that patients who have multimodality treatments also have a higher symptom burden and therefore the greatest risk of developing complex late effects. It's important that a holistic approach is taken to ensure that treatment is optimizing quality of life and to help to address the symptom burden.

There are many late consequences of treatment that pertain to specific disease types e.g., brain patients will experience long-term loss of cognitive function whereas lung patients will encounter breathlessness and rib fractures. This chapter will focus on just a few of the main tumour sites. Many patients will often experience other symptoms such as fatigue, psychological, or psychosocial issues contributing to a cluster effect of long-term consequences that is responsible for a reduced quality of life.

Head and Neck Cancers

Radiation-induced fibrosis in the head and neck area results in a loss of range of movement and associated function. For many patients, lymphoedema both externally and internally due to congestion, damage, and fibrosis of the lymphatic system contributes to a complex symptom burden, which is heightened especially if RIF and changes to the integrity of the skin are present. Such consequences lead to pain, dysphagia, hearing loss, and decrease in range of movement. Symptomatic patients may also experience trauma within the oral cavity due to oedema of the tongue and buccal mucosa. This can lead to recurrent ulcers, pain, and increased anxiety due to the fear of the cancer recurrence.

Dysphagia (due to altered structures and swallow function from the tumour), fibrotic effects, and constriction from lymphoedema can lead to long-term swallowing issues leading to the risk of aspiration and a decrease in nutritional intake.[7] Fibrosis and lymphoedema both contribute to trismus which is a chronic contraction of the TMJ muscle. This results in pain and a restriction in mouth opening, usually affecting nutrition and speech. Direct damage to the salivary glands and taste buds can cause changes in saliva production and loss or altered taste. This contributes to a chronic dry mouth and troublesome thick secretions,[8] leading to an increase of dental caries, declining nutrition, and reduced oral hygiene. Patients who experience this often have disturbed sleep contributing to higher fatigue levels.

Burning mouth syndrome is a chronic condition often enhanced by a dry mouth environment where patients experience a burning, scalding sensation often with recurrent oral thrush. Intensity and severity can fluctuate over time and throughout the day.[8] The symptom burden is so significant that some patients will develop anxiety and depression, and subsequently withdraw from socializing or other daily activities.

Osteoradionecrosis is a painful and debilitating complication of the mandible where damage to the blood supply results in exposed bone after minor trauma such as dental extractions. Treatment that incorporated the sinuses and nasal cavity can develop chronic sinusitis. This includes post-nasal drip, nasal discharge, facial pain, headaches, and dry nasal passages.

Nerve damage can lead to painful and debilitating spasms within the neck and tongue. Patients can also experience head drop syndrome due to weakness of neck extensor muscles which causes an inability for the patient to extend the neck resulting in poor posture and a flexed forward head.

Thyroid complications can occur. Hypothyroidism is common for many patients after treatment and TSH level should be monitored annually. Whilst hyperparathyroidism is less common, it can develop and lead to hypercalcaemia.

Hearing loss, balance issues, and damage to the ear often present initially as an earache and glue-like ear symptoms due to fluid collection in the middle ear. This can also be heightened if the patient is experiencing tinnitus from any adjuvant chemotherapy. Many patients will express concerns with balance and vertigo.[8]

Breast Cancer

Pain in the breast and chest wall is one of the most commonly reported effects along with change in size, shape, and how the area feels due to fibrotic changes and lymphoedema. Pain can also be a result of rib fractures and costochondritis. Critically, the psychological impact of the cancer diagnosis must always be acknowledged as a contributing factor to pain levels. In some instances, this can have a significant impact on the ability to have and maintain a physical sexual relationship, often reflecting a lack of desire related to altered body image.[9]

Decreased mobility of the shoulder along with brachial plexus neuropathy can lead to a decrease in function of the affected arm. Breathlessness associated with pulmonary fibrosis can be problematic for some patients. Similarly, respiratory capacity may have changed due to the impact of any surgeries.

Skin changes tend to be more prevalent and often present as telangiectasia, discoloration (along with less common morphea), and atrophic ulceration. Radiation-induced secondary malignancies (particularly angiosarcoma) are also recognized with an incidence of adjuvant radiotherapy-induced angiosarcoma reported as 0.05–0.3%.[10]

Pelvic Cancers

Pelvic radiation disease is defined as one or more chronic symptoms of variable complexity that patients experience as a result of pelvic radiotherapy. Given the wide range of cancers that are treated with pelvic radiotherapy many patient groups are affected including patients with colon/rectal cancers, gynaecological cancers, prostate cancer, and lymphoma. Consequences of pelvic radiotherapy affect the gastrointestinal tract, urinary tract, reproductive and sexual organs, bone, vasculature, neurological systems such as lumbosacral plexus and peripheral nerves, lymphatic system, and skin.

The Pelvic Radiation Disease Association has produced a best practice pathway for pelvic radiation disease that acts as a gold standard for the management of all of the systems affected by pelvic radiotherapy.[11] This document covers all possible known pelvic late effects such as pelvic insufficiency fractures, radiation enteropathy, bowel and bladder changes, along with the psychosocial and sexual difficulties that patients experience.

Fertility

Due to the increasing efficacy of treatment for the management of people of childbearing age there is an increasing focus on the impact of treatment on fertility. This includes robust fertility counselling prior to the commencement of treatment, wherever it is feasible to do so. Both systemic therapies and certain radiotherapy treatment can be gonadotoxic and therefore loss of fertility is a common side effect of treatment. It can be challenging to navigate these concerns particularly when individuals have yet to consider starting a family. Additionally, even if fertility preservation is offered, the trajectory of the malignancy (or the patient's systemic symptoms) may mean the intervention isn't possible. Therefore, infertility and hypogonadism, and premature ovarian insufficiency will continue to be significant consequences of treatment. More patients will require input from fertility services as the number of younger cancer survivors grows.[12]

Cardiac Toxicity

Traditionally the late impact of cancer therapy on the cardiovascular system was largely attributed to the chronic effect of the anthracyclines leading to chronic heart failure. This was initially thought to be entirely dose-density related. However, whilst reducing the maximum life-time dose of anthracyclines has reduced the impact in terms of heart failure incidence, it continues to be an issue, suggesting increased sensitivity of certain individuals to the mechanisms of toxicity. In addition to cardiac failure other late cardiac effects seen secondary to various systemic anti-cancer therapies include arrhythmias, cardiomyopathy, arterio-vascular disease, pulmonary hypertension, pericardia disease, and systemic hypertension.[13] Additionally, radiotherapy can induce valvular dysfunction if the heart is captured in the radiotherapy field.

Cardiology input in the management of these patients is essential. With optimum use of cardio-protective medications the prognosis of these conditions can be significantly improved.[13] In addition to this, in some specialist centres, specific cardio-oncology MDTs are being established with both cardiology and oncology specialist input.

Emerging Late Effects with Novel Systemic Agents

An expanding number of immunotherapies and targeted agents has led to an increasing recognition that many of these agents will also lead to chronic and complex late effects. This is becoming a focus of research. Chronic immune-related adverse events were identified in 43.2% of patients in a 2021 study.[14] Of these events, 85% lasted until the end of the study with higher rates of persisting endocrinopathies, arthralgia, ocular events, xerostomia, and cutaneous events.[14] These evolving late effects add an extra dimension to the one already identified as the toxicity paradigm caused in the acute setting by the induction of iatrogenic autoimmunity caused by checkpoint inhibitors (ICI). In addition to these treatments, newer cellular therapies such as CAR-T therapies can lead to long-term neurological and cardiac effects whilst the long-term impact of newer targeted therapies and antibody-drug conjugates is yet to be determined. As with many late effects these newer issues are best managed by an expert team and in some regions of the UK, late effects immunotherapy clinics have been established.[15,16]

Fatigue

Significant fatigue (reported as tiredness, lack of energy, and generalized aching) is common both during and after anti-cancer therapies. It is reported that between 15 and 35% of adult cancer survivors experience chronic fatigue.

Whilst comprehensive investigations can uncover often allusive but reversible causes, fatigue remains a significant issue for many patients in the long term.[17] There remains a considerable research focus on symptom management including trials of both psychological and pharmacological interventions. Chronic fatigue may lead to a considerable reduction in quality of life.[18]

Lymphoedema

Lymphoedema is the swelling and build-up of lymphatic fluid and sometimes fat. The network of drainage pathways through vessels and glands fails or is compromised by cancer treatment, termed secondary lymphoedema. Earlier stages of lymphoedema are reversible but if untreated can lead to fibrotic tissue changes and resistance to therapies. Unmanaged lymphoedema can lead to skin thickening, lymphorrhea (lymph fluid leaking through the skin), and cellulitis infections. Development of lymphoedema is increased with multi-modality treatments such as lymph node dissection followed by radiotherapy. It is a chronic condition that is usually managed conservatively with massage therapy to manually move the fluid and tight compression garments to try and prevent swelling. Cancer-related lymphoedema is dependent on the anatomical site treated; arm, hand, breast, trunk, and chest wall in breast cancer patients; legs, feet, genitals, and abdomen in pelvis cancer patients; face, larynx, and tongue in head and neck cancer patients. It can lead to poor quality of life affecting both physical and psychosocial aspects.[19,20]

Its chronic nature leaves a lasting legacy from a cancer diagnosis and treatment and could eventually impact the ability to work and cause uncontrolled pain.[21] NICE guidance[22] recommends patients should have timely access to specialist lymphoedema services; however, commissioning guidance from 2019 showed that provision is not equitable, and services have long waiting lists. Current treatments include massage therapy, compression bandaging, photobiomodulation therapy, deep oscillation treatment, and kinesio taping. In essence all these treatments are designed to manage lymphoedema rather than trying to prevent it. Prophylactic monitoring starting before treatment and early intervention may reduce the risk of chronic lymphoedema in breast cancer patients.[23]

'What Matters to You' vs 'What Is the Matter with You'

Any service designed to support the management of late consequences of treatment should be patient-centred and grounded on 'what matters to you' rather than 'what is the matter with you'. Unfortunately, many patients are left with unmet physical and psychosocial needs.[1] Why is this still the case?

Oncology services centred on diagnosis and treatment (broadly surgery, systemic anti-cancer therapies, and radiotherapy) are of little benefit to managing toxicities post-treatment. As survivorship increases, the demand on oncology services has driven strategies of accelerated discharge, stratified follow-up, and remote monitoring, designed to detect disease recurrence but not to evaluate late effects.

Accelerated discharge pathways rely on primary care physicians as first line to monitor and manage complex late effects, often supported by self-management support strategies, or on patients to recognize and understand the consequences of treatment themselves.[24] Symptoms are often unreported, or patients enter cycles of referrals between many care providers.[25] Improved models of care integrating specialist support and holistic management demonstrate clear benefits in terms of symptom support and financial viability.[7] Access to non-oncological specialities depending on the profile of late side-effects is required and the number of specialities this includes is ever growing as cancer treatment modalities continue to diversify and late effects experiences are increasingly recognized.

Care needs to be accessible and appropriate, and referrals to local services efficient and co-ordinated. To achieve this a "single point of access" can help optimize care from non-oncology specialisms and improve the overall patient experience. Nurse or Allied Health Professional (AHP)-led follow-up clinics have been shown to be effective for pelvic radiotherapy patients.[26,27] All models of late effects services must reflect the needs of people affected by cancer from 'legacy' patients treated many years ago to those just starting on treatment.

Multi-Disciplinary (MDT) Working

Managing late effects is a team effort extending beyond the remit of the oncology department and secondary care. Established late effects clinics are often run by a single member of staff expected to cover all anatomical sites and diagnoses safely and effectively over extended time frames. This member of staff is often a nurse or AHP rather than a medic, and often inadequately trained as late effects are not widely included in any oncology curriculum.

Management options such as surgery for late effects are often excluded due to poor healing or a lack of evidence. Expertise from beyond the oncology setting is warranted as some treatments, such as urinary incontinence medication, mirror those of patients who have not had cancer treatments.[28] MDT working is required at a local level to ensure patients can access care close to home, regionally where larger centres have specialized services, or nationally for expert advice. National engagement is essential for legacy patients who may have moved location and received care from a wide network of providers over a long period of time. As well as benefitting decision making and patient care, the MDT also allows feedback about late effects to oncology and acute care teams. Prospective management of late effects can benefit from MDT working with shared knowledge and discussion detecting late effects earlier and providing better interventions. The MDT can provide an early feedback loop for information that is currently only reported in trials often many years after treatment or not shared at all.

MDT working provides a mechanism for discussion, safety, and peer support in decision making. It provides patients with options that might not have been available locally through service development and trials. The traditional cancer MDT was devised to provide personalized treatment for patients; the late effects MDT should provide holistic personalized care beyond treatment.[7]

References

1. Maher J et al. Implementation of nationwide cancer survivorship plans: experience from the UK. *J Cancer Policy*. 2018;15:76–81.
2. Schmidt ME et al. Quality of life, problems, and needs of disease-free breast cancer survivors 5 years after diagnosis. *Qual Life Res*. 2018;27(8):2077–2086.
3. Schmidt ME et al. Late effects, long term problems and unmet needs of cancer survivors. *Int J Cancer* 2022;151:1280–1290.
4. Hashmi SK et al. National institutes of health blood and marrow transplant late effects initiative: The healthcare delivery working group report. *Biol Blood Marrow Transplant*. 2017;23(5):717–725.
5. Bryant AK et al. Trends in radiation therapy amongst cancer survivors in the United States, 2000–2030. *Cancer Epidemiol Biomarkers Prev*. 2017;26:963–970.
6. Purkayastha A et al. Radiation fibrosis syndrome: The evergreen menace of radiotherapy. *Asia-Pacific J Oncol Nursing*. 2019;6:238–245.
7. Muls AC et al. The holistic management of consequences of cancer treatment by a gastrointestinal and nutrition team: a financially viable approach to an enormous problem? *Clin Med*. 2016;16(3):240–246.
8. Brook I. Late side effects of radiation treatment for head and neck cancer. *Radiat Oncol J*. 2020;38(2):84–92.
9. Wallgren A. Late effects of radiotherapy in the treatment of breast cancer. *Acta Oncologica*. 1991;31:237–242.
10. Suzuki Y et al. Recurring radiation-induced angiosarcoma of the breast that was treated with paclitaxel chemotherapy: a case report. *Surg Case Rep*. 2020;16;6(1):25.
11. Pelvic Disease Association UK, Best Practice Pathway Toolkit [internet], available at: https://www.prda.org.uk/wp-content/uploads/2022/09/PRDA_Best-Practice-Pathway_Toolkit.pdf (accessed Aug 2023).
12. Rodriguez-Wallberg KA et al. The late effects of cancer treatment on female fertility and the current status of fertility preservation—a narrative review. *Life*. 2023;13(5):1195.
13. Lon A et al, ESC Guidelines on cardio-oncology developed in collaboration with the European Hematology Association (EHA), the European Society for Therapeutic Radiology and Oncology (ESTRO) and the International Cardio-Oncology Society (IC-OS): developed by the task force on cardio-oncology of the European Society of Cardiology (ESC). *European Heart J*. 2022;43:4229–2361.
14. Patrinely JR Jr et al. Chronic immune-related adverse events following adjuvant anti-PD-1 therapy for high-risk resected melanoma. *JAMA Oncol*. 2021;7(5):744–748.
15. Guinan TJ et al. The impact of an immuno-oncology service at a regional cancer centre based in the north west of the UK. *Br J Nurs*. 2022;21;31(8):414–420.
16. Oxtoby K. Late effects of cancer treatment: what nurses need to know. *Cancer Nurs Practice*. 2023;22:6–8.

17. Bower JE. Cancer-related fatigue – mechanisms, risk factors, and treatments. *Nat Rev Clin Oncol.* 2014;11(10):597–609.

18. Reinertsen KV et al. Chronic fatigue in adult cancer survivors. *Tidsskriftet Den Norske Legeforening.* 2017;1:1–7.

19. Morgan PA et al. Health-related quality of life with lymphoedema: a review of the literature. *Int Wound J.* 2005;2(1):47–62.

20. Bowman C et al. Living with leg lymphedema: developing a novel model of quality lymphedema care for cancer survivors. *J Cancer Surviv.* 2021;15(1):140–150.

21. Moffatt CJ et al. Lymphoedema: an underestimated health problem. *QJM.* 2003;96(10):731–738.

22. NICE. Early and locally advanced breast cancer: diagnosis and management, NG101, 2018, updated 2024, available at: https://www.nice.org.uk/guidance/ng101.

23. Rafn BS, et al. Prospective surveillance for breast cancer-related arm lymphedema: a systematic review and meta-analysis. *J Clin Oncol.* 2022;40(9):1009–1026.

24. Dineen-Griffin S et al. Helping patients help themselves: a systematic review of self-management support strategies in primary health care practice. *PLoS One.* 2019;14(8):e0220116.

25. Macmillan Cancer Support. Cured – but at what cost? Long-term consequences of cancer and its treatment [internet], 2013, available at: https://www.macmillan.org.uk/dfsmedia/1a6f235 37f7f4519bb0cf14c45b2a629/14614-10061/cured-but-at-what-cost-summary-report-july-2013.

26. Faithfull S et al. Evaluation of nurse-led follow up for patients undergoing pelvic radiotherapy. *Br J Cancer* 2001;85:1853–1864.

27. Ludlow H et al. Late gastrointestinal effects of pelvic radiation: a nurse-led service. *Br J Nursing* 2017;26:S15–S22.

28. Ritchey M et al. Late effects on the urinary bladder in patients treated for cancer in childhood: a report from the children's oncology group. *Pediatr Blood Cancer.* 2009;52(4):439–446.

5

Patient Optimization and Rehabilitation

Victoria Jones, Malcolm Brown, Laura Miller, Tasha Critchlow, and Ben Heyworth

Introduction

The National Cancer Research Institute (NCRI) estimates that by 2030, four million people in the UK will be living with the long-term effects of cancer. Managing this patient population poses a unique challenge, with the emphasis placed on improving the quality of survivorship and offsetting cancer-related toxicities. Several supportive therapies can assist during this phase, with physical activity (PA), emotional and psychological distress, spiritual care, dietetics, and smoking cessation discussed within this chapter.

Physical Activity

In recent years, PA (movement involving skeletal muscles resulting in energy expenditure) or indeed exercise training (planned, structured, and repetitive activity for physical fitness) has gained recognition as an effective therapy in cancer care. This area of research, coined 'exercise oncology', has increased exponentially with accumulating evidence-based findings advocating exercise training throughout the cancer continuum.[1]

Prehabilitation encompasses the prescription of healthy lifestyle interventions to prepare patients for cancer treatment (e.g., surgery). Essentially, this personalized intervention empowers patients to optimize their physical and mental health, facilitate treatment tolerance, and maximize resilience to treatment-related toxicities. Interventions should commence as early as possible but can prove effective with as little as two weeks of exercise training.[2] Patients not prescribed prehabilitation usually deteriorate more rapidly and are more likely to be affected by treatment side effects. Of course, there are circumstances when prehabilitation is not possible, but many clinicians now consider prehabilitation essential to the whole cancer pathway.[3]

During and following treatment, into survivorship, patients often experience numerous disease- and/or treatment-related toxicities, that ultimately impact health-related quality of life (HRQoL). These adverse outcomes include cardiotoxicity, lymphoedema, sexual dysfunction, incontinence, anxiety/depression, and fatigue, to name but a few.

Unsurprisingly, anti-cancer treatment and associated toxicities markedly impair physical fitness, increasing the risk of developing comorbidities (e.g., cardiovascular disease, sarcopenia) and decreasing the quality and length of survival. Encouragingly, exercise training has been utilized as both an adjuvant and rehabilitation strategy to reduce the

DOI: 10.1201/9781003369912-11

consequences of conventional therapies. Exercise training has proved to be a safe, feasible, and effective therapeutic strategy in disease management, invoking several physiological and psychological benefits that can prevent inevitable decline and attenuate the severity of toxicities. Aerobic (i.e., brisk walking; cycling; swimming), resistance (i.e., dumbbells; resistance bands; body weight), and mindfulness-based (i.e., Tai Chi, yoga) interventions, either in isolation or combined, have proved effective for a variety of cancers.[4–6] The benefits of exercise training[7] include:

- Improved cardiovascular fitness
- Improved body composition/fat loss
- Improved metabolism/glucose control
- Improved immunity/anti-inflammatory
- Improved sleep
- Improved fatigue
- Improved mental health/decreased anxiety and depression
- Reduced risk of recurrent disease
- Improved survival (epidemiological evidence)
- Enhanced recovery/post-treatment complications
- Reduced length of hospital stays
- Reduced risk of other diseases/sarcopenia
- Improved quality of life

Many of the accrued benefits of exercise training greatly impact quality of life in survivorship and provide important prognostic and predictive information. Likewise, capturing subjective and personal experiences provides a comprehensive, holistic perspective on the impact of exercise training in treatment tolerance. However, there remain numerous debates in this area of research.

Topical Debates in Exercise Oncology

Little consensus exists regarding the optimal exercise dose (e.g., duration; intensity) to be prescribed and how this varies with differential diagnoses.[7,8] The overwhelming majority of evidence advocates exercise training during and following treatment, although the heterogeneity of exercise prescription, assessment methods, different patient populations, and healthcare settings creates a level of uncertainty. Further research should seek to clarify the optimal dose; however simply getting patients who are sedentary active is a good starting point.

Likewise, the level of supervision and the site of delivery remain a topic of debate[9] Supervised exercise, under the guidance of a qualified professional, tends to be the most effective.[10] However, supervised exercise is a resource-intensive model, undoubtably unsustainable in most global health systems, including the NHS, facing economic and staffing challenges.[11]

Home-based (perhaps digitally supported) exercise may prove a suitable alternative, increasing accessibility and flexibility to integrate exercise around lifestyle and treatment toxicities (e.g., the Safe-Fit Trial[12]). Alternatively, refining and utilizing referral pathways to either community-based exercise initiatives (e.g., Macmillan Move More) or clinical exercise trials could improve equality in access.[13] Regardless of the delivery method, exercise training could prove a cost-effective option;[14] however, this needs to be demonstrated in practice.

Next, the majority of evidence to date has been assembled from the most prevalent cancers (e.g., breast, prostate), in patients with curable disease or during survivorship, creating a level of bias. Only recently has attention been diverted to advanced cancers – meaning this evidence base is limited. Perhaps this move is connected to improved survival rates with advanced cancers (e.g., prostate cancer) or the conceptualization of 'metastatic survivorship' and recognition that exercise training could improve the quality of palliative care and potentially survival.[15]

Whilst research into advanced cancers has many complexities, it is undoubtedly worthwhile. The benefits previously mentioned extend to advanced cancers[16–21] and these intangibles may be crucial when further treatment is required. The supportive oncology MDT should consider proactively discussing suitability for exercise training, 'championing' exercise during consultations, and providing information around the benefits of being active, including signposting and formal referral pathways.

Finally, the anti-tumour impact of exercise training remains to be determined. Preclinical research is the only setting to have shown exercise training can reprogramme the systemic milieu and improve conditions within the tumour microenvironment (e.g., improved tumour perfusion; decreased hypoxia; decreased tumour growth).[22] Moreover, exercise training has been reported to improve the efficacy of conventional therapy in mice;[23] however, translational research in humans is severely limited and further research attention is warranted.

Barriers to Moving More

Despite accumulating robust evidence regarding the positive effects and safety of exercise, few survivors meet recommended guidelines. A recent systematic review of 4000 cancer survivors revealed the most common barriers to exercise are treatment-related side effects, lack of time, and fatigue. A lack of information, education, and support is also a significant barrier, particularly the type and intensity of exercise that is safest or most effective.[24]

Obviously, cancer-specific barriers also present significant obstacles to participation (e.g., stoma; lymphoedema) and each requires considered personalization, based on individual circumstances. Removing such barriers is essential to encourage PA. Identifying the most prominent allows clinicians to support, educate, and refer onto community-based initiatives.

Within the UK, Macmillan Move More is perhaps the most recognized referral programme. This scheme educates people living with cancer on the benefits of PA and enables them to become and stay active. This is achieved through supervised, community-based classes, information, and support to empower behavioural change. Thus, this referral programme and others alike (e.g., RENEW[25]) are strong facilitators for overcoming barriers faced during survivorship.

Emotional and Psychological Distress

Emotional distress associated with a cancer diagnosis may take on a myriad of forms; it could be understood as a period of grief and loss, or as a significant change of role going from being healthy to being "sick" and all that entails.[26] Furthermore, people living with cancer can be stigmatized and wonder "why me" with regards to their diagnosis.[27]

Cancer diagnoses can provoke profound anxiety in the face of uncertainty around response to treatment and cancer course, whilst the process of being investigated for and treated for cancer can be traumatic, leading to cancer-related post-traumatic stress disorder (CR-PTSD).[28] Given the heightened opportunity for emotional distress, appropriate screening is the first step in ensuring people living with cancer are adequately supported in an individualized fashion.

Screening Tools and the Role of Supportive Oncology

Tools like the Distress Thermometer (DT), which is endorsed by the National Comprehensive Cancer Network in the USA, have been used across different clinical settings to screen for emotional distress in people living with cancer.[29] The DT is accessible as it can be administered by any health professional who has undertaken appropriate training.[30] It asks people to rate their emotional distress and includes a 39-item problem list grouped according to practical, family, emotional, spiritual/religious, and physical issues.[29] Though the DT cannot accurately identify anxiety or depressive disorders, if moderate to severe distress is identified this can prompt oncology professionals to consider undertaking further screening for anxiety and depression (for example, using the GAD-7 and PHQ-9 tools respectively).[31,32]

Furthermore, statistical analysis shows that emotional, physical, and spiritual items identified on the problem list are significantly associated with moderate-severe distress, highlighting the importance of the joined up supportive oncology MDT approach.[29] Barriers to the implementation of distress-screening tools include lack of privacy, lack of training for staff, and lack of infrastructure to support screening.[33,34] To capture the individualized needs of people living with cancer in more depth, structured Holistic Needs Assessments are useful though implementation is heterogeneous across different countries and settings.[35]

The use of screening tools allows early detection of issues and personalized support can be offered proactively, potentially halting symptoms from deteriorating further. The question of who is responsible for this screening highlights the complex interplay between areas of cancer care. Though every healthcare contact is an opportunity to explore psychological symptoms and enable early identification of issues, psycho-oncology departments offer more specialized input including counselling and other talking therapies.

A collaborative approach between oncology and psycho-oncology departments has proven fruitful at the Princess Margaret Cancer Centre (PMCC) in Toronto, where there is more than 70% uptake of the distress screening throughout the hospital. At PMCC, a bespoke Distress Assessment and Response Tool (DART) was developed to meet the state symptom screening requirements for cancer care, whilst also including in-depth screening incorporating specific measures of anxiety, depression, physical symptoms, and practical needs. Clinic patients are directed to complete the DART in waiting areas prior to appointments, with both online and paper copies available. Patients with high DART scores are further assessed by specialized oncology nurses to guide further intervention as required.[33]

DART evaluation showed increased teamwork amongst staff with no detrimental impact on workload or clinic duration, and patients reported that DART improved communication with their teams and reported greater satisfaction with emotional support received.

Effective Interventions

Once distress has been identified, interventions can be tailored to the patient and their needs. Non-pharmacological interventions such as supportive listening and signposting to services such as complementary therapies are also effective.[36] Other condition-specific interventions such as eye movement desensitization and reprocessing (EMDR) therapy for cancer-related PTSD, anxiety management skills such as mindfulness, or cognitive behavioural therapy for depression are also effective.[37,38] The supportive oncology MDT can lead this support, whilst also referring on to local psycho-oncology teams for more specialized input if required, though long waiting lists may be a barrier to accessing this support.

At the Princess Margaret Centre, implementation of DART was not followed by a huge increase in referrals to psycho-oncology, but instead prompted more frequent assessments in clinic and recognition that alleviation of one symptom, for example pain, may improve symptoms related to emotional distress without need for further referral.[33]

In addition to non-pharmacological measures, medication has an important role in identified mental illness such as anxiety or depression. Any potential benefit needs to be carefully weighed up against side effects, and the length of time needed for the medication to take effect.

Throughout this process, collaborating with the patient is key. Supportive oncology plays a crucial role in enabling people to take responsibility for decisions around their care, working together with them to help navigate the emotional distress they may be experiencing.[39]

Spiritual Care

Not every distressed patient requires counselling or therapy. Cancer challenges meaning and relationships in the patient's life and forces revaluation of the world around them. Here we refer to a spiritual 'realm' where an individual is readjusting values and beliefs. The importance of this existential reshuffle has been noted as essential for general wellbeing, making decisions around care, and even the healing process.[40]

Spirituality plays an important part in the adjustment process for a patient with atheistic worldview as much as for a patient with religious beliefs. Using the definition of spirituality suggested by Elkins and colleagues,[41] we can concentrate on four main areas of spiritual need: Self, others, nature/life, and the ultimate. Let's take Anne's story, created from the experiences of several patients, to illustrate this process using the spiritual assessment tool developed by Nolan.[42]

Anne has been told that the latest intervention did not work, and a new care plan would begin. She became very tearful. Her medical team recognized spiritual distress and knew they were not best placed to address it. A chaplain was called in.

Death was not Anne's greatest fear. She was more concerned about what was happening to her (SELF), her body, her ability to eat and taste, the way things around her smelled, her independence; could she still play the piano now that her fingers were numb from chemo? "What's the point of prolonging life if I am like this?"

(OTHERS) Anne was especially upset because she was worried that she wouldn't see her 3-week old grandson grow up. "He will never know me!" She worried about her husband. "How will he cope? And we had so many plans."

(NATURE and LIFE) Anne longed to sit in her garden. Being in the hospital oppressed her and she felt trapped. Her walls were covered with prints of Monet and four vases with flowers crowded her bed. She was also worried about her business and tried to continue working whenever she could.

(The ULTIMATE) And what will happen to her when she dies? She was brought up a Christian but "has become very practical" and left all of that behind. "I don't know what I believe in anymore!" She wanted to plan her funeral, asked for her hymnal to be brought, and spent hours reading poetry.

Subsequent conversations with Anne revealed the importance of many spiritual factors that influenced her decisions about medical treatment and overall quality of life. She chose to attend Ash Wednesday service and the familiar liturgy helped her to reflect on her mortality. A piano in the chapel was left unlocked so that Anne could play whilst she still could. She found it helpful to speak about her changing body and place in the family as "only an observer now". She decided to write to her grandson a few letters full of memories so that they didn't disappear with her. She planned her funeral and found comfort in knowing that the chaplain who knew her well would take the service, even if the end came several years later. Anne voiced her concerns and wishes to her medical team and knew she had been heard.

The medical team were able to identify Anne's spiritual distress and refer her to a chaplain for assessment of her needs and support in liaising with her treating team. The role of chaplains in supportive oncology interdisciplinary teams is well-recognized in the UK.[43] Taken seriously, patients can process and adjust to the illness in line with what is important to them. There is evidence to suggest that illness can result in positive transformation in some patients. They take control of their lives and prioritize what really matters.[44]

Diet and Nutrition

Cancer incidence is rising, with about 40% of these cases thought to be preventable with changes to diet, reduced alcohol consumption, increased physical activity, and maintaining a healthy weight. Our understanding of the interplay between diet, lifestyle, and

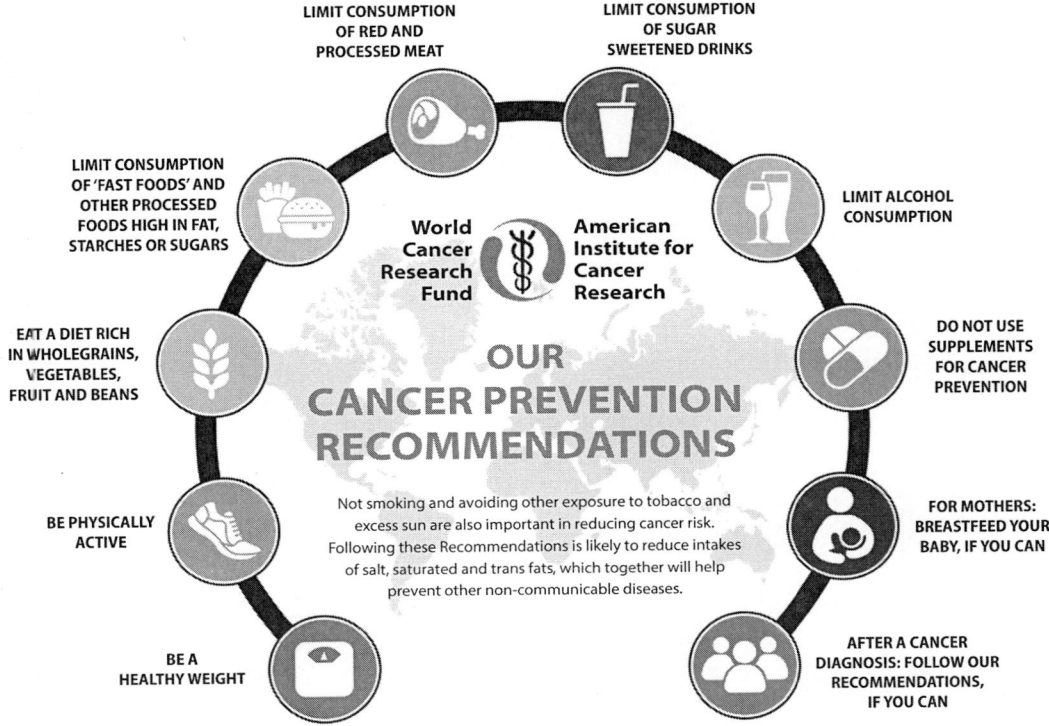

FIGURE 5.1
Diet and lifestyle recommendations for cancer prevention (reproduced with permission from ref 45).

cancer risk has increased significantly in part due to collective global research efforts. International research collaborations such as the Global Cancer Update Programme (CUP Global[45]) have identified dietary risk factors in 17 cancers informing global public health policy (Figure 5.1). However, our understanding of the impacts of diet on rarer cancers and certain populations remains limited.

Nutritional Risk

The relationship between nutrition and cancer is complex and optimizing our understanding to improve interventions has been confounded by a lack of agreed terminology and diagnostic criteria.[46] The UN defines malnutrition as a "deficiency (undernutrition), excess (overnutrition including obesity), or imbalance in a person's intake or use of energy and/or nutrients."[47] This definition portrays three categories of nutritional risk. Those who are undernourished, overweight/obese, and those with micro- or macronutrient deficiencies. Each should be considered by the supportive oncology team. The under-reporting of nutritional comorbidities is further compounded by poor implementation of nutrition guidelines[48] and limited health professional knowledge and training on nutrition.[49,50]

Malnutrition

Malnutrition is often associated with wasting and underweight, however this underestimates micronutrient deficiencies and the impact on people who are overweight or obese. Incidence of malnutrition ranges between 30 and 90% (by validated screening tools) with up to 20% of people with cancer dying from malnutrition before their malignancy. It negatively impacts the survival, hospital admissions, quality of life, morbidity, mortality, and the healthcare costs of people with cancer.[51,52]

As such supportive oncology teams should facilitate routine nutrition screening at the earliest opportunity and repeat throughout treatment using a validated tool.[53,54] For those identified at risk a further comprehensive assessment using a validated instrument, i.e., pgSGA, or process, i.e., dietetic care process, by a trained professional such as a dietician is required.[55,56]

The Global Leaders in Malnutrition (GLIM) have proposed diagnostic criteria for malnutrition that look beyond body mass index (BMI): They recommend a combination of observable (phenotypic) and disease-related measures (etiologic),[57] detailing the prognostic complexity of cancer-associated malnutrition, including cancer-mediated inflammatory changes (cancer cachexia). Figure 5.2 shares these criteria and proposes assessment strategies supportive oncology teams may consider.

For patients with reduced intake or malnutrition, dietary interventions should be personalized based on activity levels, preferences (informed by faith or beliefs), symptoms, and comorbidities.[58] Professionals should consider encouraging a diverse range of foods and managing potential micronutrient deficiencies with advanced strategies including enteral feeding. Accurately determining energy and protein demands is complex and targets should be realistic, aligning to the stage of the disease and potential symptom burden, and adjusted to prevent overfeeding (preventing obesity). Nutritional interventions that facilitate muscle maintenance – protein, amino acids, omega-3, vitamin D, creatinine – are key to supporting improved outcomes irrespective of body type[59] and should be considered as part of a multimodal intervention.

Obesity: Challenges and Opportunities

The impact of being overweight or obese on cancer treatment outcomes remains inconclusive, conferring differential survival and morbidity risks dependent on type of cancer and stage of treatment. Increased adiposity (fat) is associated with risk of developing several cancers possibly due to chronic low-level inflammation.

Supportive oncology teams should avoid preconceptions that people who have cancer and are overweight/obese are well nourished and do not require nutritional care. Stigma and inadequate nutrition screening can lead to systemic under-identification of nutritional risk in this population. Hormone therapies, inactivity, cancer-related inflammation, and reduced dietary intake can result in altered body composition, leading to a higher fat to muscle ratio, a state known as sarcopenic obesity. Sarcopenic obesity is independently associated with poor cancer outcomes.

1 or more phenotypic criteria AND 1 or more etiologic criteria

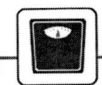

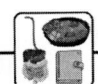

| Unintentional weight loss | Low Body Mass Index | Reduced muscle mass | | Reduced food intake or assimilation | Presence of cancer related inflammation |

Unintentional weight loss

Measure:
• Percentage (%) weight loss

How:
• What was your normal weight 6 months ago?
• Is weight loss unintentional: Have you been trying to lose weight i.e. dieting in this time?
• **BMI:** (Current weight (kg)/weight 6 months ago (Kg)) x 100

Criteria:
• >5% within past 6 months, or >10% beyond 6 months

Considerations:
• Is oedema/ascites accounted for?
• Know the evidence: What % weight loss is significant in your cancer group?

Low Body Mass Index

Measure:
• BMI (kg/m2)

How:
• Weight (kg)/ height2 (m2)

Criteria:
• Under 70yrs: < 20 kg/m2
• Over 70 yrs: < 22 kg/m2
Asian populations:
• Under 70 yrs: <18.5 kg/m2
• Over 70 yrs <20 kg/m2

Considerations:
• Does the weight and height appear realistic.
• Is oedema and ascites accounted for.

Reduced muscle mass

Measure: Changes in muscle mass measured using a validated method

How:
• **Low cost:** Calf or mid-arm muscle circumference
• **Imaging:** DEXA, CT, MRI, BIA & ultrasound
• **Indirect measures:** Handgrip strength

Criteria:
• Use consensus recommendations i.e. EWGSOP; FNIH and AWGS

Considerations:
• Use population specific cut offs (i.e. sex and ethnicity)

+

Reduced food intake or assimilation

Measure: Change in dietary intake (food diary, 24hr recall) and symptom burden (i.e. stool chart, steatorrhea)

Criteria:
• **1 or more of the following**
• <50% of energy requirements for >1 wk
• Any reduction for >2 wks
• Any chronic GI condition that adversely impacts food assimilation or absorption i.e. obstruction, high output stoma

Considerations:
• Routine monitoring of symptoms that may affect food intake or absorption

Presence of cancer related inflammation

Measure: Systemic inflammation, informed by cancer disease burden

How:
• modified Glasgow prognostic score,
• Inflammatory markers i.e.
• CRP

Criteria: Suspected presence or absence of cancer related inflammation.

Considerations:
• Severity of disease burden
• Response to treatment
• Are there any other causes i.e. infection.

Severity based on phenotypic criteria

1 or more phenotypic criteria	Weight loss (%)	Low body mass index (kg/m2)	Reduced Muscle Mass
Stage 1/Moderate Malnutrition	5-10% within the past 6 mths, or 10-20% beyond 6 mths	<20 if <70 yr, <22 if ≥70 yr	Mild to moderate deficit (per validated assessment methods)
Stage 2/Severe Malnutrition	> 10% within the past 6 mths or > 20% beyond 6 mths	<18.5 if <70 yr, <20 if ≥70 yr	Severe deficit (per validated assessment methods)

Diagnostic terminology

• Chronic disease with inflammation (or cancer cachexia)
• Chronic disease with minimal or no perceived inflammation
• Acute disease or injury with severe inflammation
• Starvation including hunger/food shortage associated with socio-economic or environmental factors

Micronutrient deficiencies

• Where prolonged nutritional deficits (intake or malabsorption) are observed:
  ○ Monitor for vitamin and mineral deficiencies
  ○ Screen, treat and monitor for refeeding syndrome where appropriate
• Be aware of drug-nutrient interactions

FIGURE 5.2
Consensus diagnostic criteria for malnutrition and considerations for supportive oncology teams (adapted from data in refs 52 and 57]. DEXA, dual energy X-ray absorptiometry; BIA, bioelectrical impedance analysis; CT, computerized tomography; EWGSOP, European Working Group on Sarcopenia in Older People; FNIH, Foundation of National Institutes of Health initiative; AWGS, Asian Working Group on Sarcopenia.

Including strategies to measure muscle loss as part of nutrition screening and assessment practices is recommended. Strategies used will depend on equipment, cost, and time but include imaging (e.g., CT sliceometry, MRI, DEXA) and low-cost measures (e.g., calf-circumference, triceps skin fold). Alongside this there is also a lack of research on the impact of managed weight loss before or during treatment on clinical outcomes. Strategies such as time-restricted eating or intermittent fasting are gaining interest but well-designed studies to inform practice recommendations are lacking. Those wishing to follow restrictive diets for weight loss purposes during active treatment should be monitored closely to mitigate nutrient deficiencies.

Smoking Cessation

Decades of research suggest that stopping smoking can have a significant impact on clinical outcomes for people affected by cancer.[60–66] The clinical benefits of smoking cessation are well documented, and include a reduction in the risk of recurrence, improved efficacy of cancer treatments, and reduction of the likelihood and severity of acute side effects and late consequences of treatment.[66] There is significant evidence to suggest that individuals enjoy improvements to their mental health and mood, physical fitness, financial wellbeing, and overall quality of life.[66]

Smoking rates across the world vary considerably. In the UK, smoking rates have been consistently dropping for decades, with current epidemiology suggesting a rate of between 12.7% and 14.9% (equating to around 6 million adults).[63] This drop is largely as a result of anti-tobacco campaigns and improvements with regard to education on the harms of tobacco smoking.

Managing Tobacco Dependence

Quitting can be hard and tobacco dependence should be considered a chronic condition with a high likelihood of relapse. It is likely that patients will need targeted, long-term support both from the supportive oncology MDT, primary care, and specialist smoking cessation professionals.[60] Supportive oncology MDTs should be encouraged to take an active role in supporting patients who wish to stop smoking.

Challenges around translating evidence-based research into practical support within supportive oncology MDTs include ingrained patient and staff attitudes towards smoking and smoking cessation and lack of knowledge or training around what interventions might be effective.[61] Care may also have to be effectively coordinated between secondary and tertiary settings and primary and community-based providers. Smokers are 4 times more likely to quit if they are signposted to specialist support; however, this may not be readily available in every geography.[66]

A "Harm-Reduction" Approach

Pharmacological interventions for smoking cessation focus on nicotine replacement therapies (NRT) which reduce withdrawal symptoms and are often available "over the counter" in the form of patches, gums, and lozenges. Other NRT interventions include inhalers and nasal sprays, the availability of which will vary from country to country. Varenicline is a nicotine receptor partial agonist that reduces withdrawal symptoms by blocking nicotine receptors. Similarly, bupropion is a dopamine and norepinephrine reuptake inhibitor with nicotine receptor antagonist properties that reduce cravings.

Approaches to non-pharmacological interventions for smoking cessation can include 1:1 or group support from trained counsellors, which could be conducted face to face or remotely. However, this approach may be expensive especially if offered in combination with drug therapies, and there may long waiting lists for services.

Using pharmacological and talking therapies in combination can increase the chances of successfully quitting and combining long-acting NRT (patch) with short-acting NRT (e.g., gum, lozenge) can also improve outcomes.[60] However, a word of caution – some studies have suggested that for every 100 patients who attempt to quit with a combination of therapies (excluding vapes/e-cigarettes), only four to seven smokers will succeed in the long term.[67] Despite this challenge, a consensus for a "harm-reduction approach" amongst smoking cessation professionals has been reached.

E-cigarette use, or vaping, continues to grow in popularity across the world. Eight per cent of Americans report having smoked e-cigarettes or "vaped" on a weekly basis – consistent with the figures Gallup recorded in 2019 (8%) and 2021 (6%) but nearly double the number from three years previous.[68] The evidence that vaping is a safer alternative to smoking cigarettes as part of a harm-reduction approach to smoking cessation is persuasive but there may be undocumented risks associated with vaping in the longer term.

Does switching to a vape help people manage their tobacco dependence? A study conducted in the Netherlands suggests that vaping may help smokers who aren't able to quit reduce the number of cigarettes smoked per day for up to six months – the duration of the study – but other studies suggest that the use of e-cigarettes only marginally improves the number of successful quit attempts in the longer term.[69]

"Very Brief Advice" and CURE

All healthcare professionals can be trained to offer "very brief advice" (VBA) around smoking cessation. VBA is a simple 30-second intervention that establishes readiness to quit and offers signposting advice to services where the individual can find support. VBA protocols were designed in the United Kingdom and have been widely adopted in that country. A study undertaken by the University of Plymouth investigated whether VBA interventions could be effective in Crete, Kyrgyzstan, Uganda, and Vietnam and the results suggested VBA interventions could be adapted to low- and middle-income countries but required local adaptations to the training resources to ensure cultural appropriateness and sensitivity.[65]

VBA is a simple and safe intervention that all healthcare professionals should consider adopting in everyday practice. In Greater Manchester in the UK, the CURE protocol has been set up specifically to 'medicalize' tobacco addiction and reduce the stigma that is associated with smoking as a lifestyle choice that may impact the likeliness of a successful quit attempt. This ensures that curing addiction becomes part of the care package offered within secondary care. The programme aims to identify all active smokers and offer take-home nicotine replacement therapy for a minimum of two weeks following discharge.[62] Supportive oncology MDTs should consider integrating an approach like CURE to help people living with cancer who may wish to quit.

References

1. Jones LW, Alfano CM. Exercise-oncology research: past, present, and future. *Acta Oncology.* 2013;52:195–215.
2. Liu Z et al. Two-week multimodal prehabilitation program improves perioperative functional capability in patients undergoing thoracoscopic lobectomy for lung cancer: a randomized controlled trial. *Anesth Analg.* 2020;131(3):840–849.
3. NIHR Cancer and Nutrition Collaboration, Royal College of Anaesthetics, Macmillan Cancer Support. Prehabilitation for people with cancer: principles and guidance for prehabilitation within the management and support of people with cancer [internet], 2020, available at: https://cdn.macmillan.org.uk/dfsmedia/1a6f23537f7f4519bb0cf14c45b2a629/1532-source/prehabilitation-for-people-with-cancer-tcm9-353994.
4. Mustian KM et al. Exercise recommendations for cancer-related fatigue, cognitive impairment, sleep problems, depression, pain, anxiety, and physical dysfunction: a review. *Oncol Hematol Rev.* 2012;8(2):81–88.
5. Buffart LM et al. Effects and moderators of exercise on quality of life and physical function in patients with cancer: an individual patient data meta-analysis of 34 RCTs. *Cancer Treat Rev.* 2017;52:91–104.
6. Segal R et al. Exercise for people with cancer: a systematic review. *Curr Oncol* 2017;24(4):e290–e315.
7. Campbell KL et al. Exercise guidelines for cancer survivors: consensus statement from international multidisciplinary roundtable. *Med Sci Sports Exerc.* 2019;51(11):2375–2390.
8. Kenfield SA et al. Physical activity and survival after prostate cancer diagnosis in the health professional: follow-up study. *J Clin Oncol.* 2011;29:726–732.
9. Kraemer MB et al. Home-based, supervised, and mixed exercise intervention on functional capacity and quality of life of colorectal cancer patients: a meta-analysis. *Sci Rep.* 2022;12;2471.
10. Westphal T et al. Supervised versus autonomous exercise training in breast cancer patients: a multicenter randomized clinical trial. *Cancer Med.* 2018;7(12):5962–5972.
11. Buchan J et al. *Rising Pressure: The NHS workforce Challenge – Workforce Profile and Trends of the NHS in England [internet].* The Health Foundation, 2017, available at: https://www.health.org .uk/publications/rising-pressure-the-nhs-workforce-challenge.
12. Grimmett C et al. SafeFit trial: virtual clinics to deliver a multimodal intervention to improve psychological and physical well-being in people with cancer: protocol of a COVID-19 targeted non-randomised phase III trial. *BMJ Open.* 2021;11:e048175.
13. National Institute for Health and Care Excellence. *Prostate Cancer: Diagnosis and Management.* NICE Guideline 131 [internet], 2019, available at: www.nice.org.uk/guidance/ng131.
14. Gubler-Gut BE et al. Cost-effectiveness of physical activity interventions in cancer survivors of developed countries: a systematic review. *J Cancer Survivorship.* 2021;15(6):961–975.
15. Lai-Kwon J et al. Evolving landscape of metastatic cancer survivorship – reconsidering clinical care, policy, and research priorities for the modern era. *J Clin Oncol.* 2023;41(18):3304–3310.
16. Cormie P et al. Safety and efficacy of resistance exercise in prostate cancer patients with bone metastases. *Prostate Cancer Prostatic Dis.* 2013;16:328–335.
17. Galvao DA et al. Exercise preserves physical function in prostate cancer patients with bone metastases. *Med Sci Sports Exerc.* 2018;50:393–399.
18. Kenfield SA et al. Feasibility, safety, and acceptability of a remotely monitored exercise pilot CHAMP: a clinical trial of high-intensity aerobic and resistance exercise for metastatic castrate-resistant prostate cancer. *Cancer Med.* 2021;10:8058–8070.
19. Hanson ED et al. Feasibility of home-based exercise training in men with metastatic castration-resistant prostate cancer. *Prostate Cancer Prostatic Dis.* 2023;26(2):302–308.
20. Kim JS et al. Exercise in advanced prostate cancer elevates myokine levels and suppresses in-vitro cell growth. *Prostate Cancer Prostatic Dis.* 2022;25:86–92.
21. Brown M et al. 2023. Feasibility of home-based exercise training during adjuvant treatment for metastatic castrate-resistant prostate cancer patients treated with an androgen receptor pathway inhibitor (EXACT). *Support Care Cancer.* 2023;31(7):442.

22. Betof AS et al. Modulation of murine breast tumor vascularity, hypoxia, and chemotherapeutic response by exercise. *J Natl Cancer Inst.* 2015;107(5):djv040.

23. Dufresne S et al. Exercise training improves radiotherapy efficiency in a murine model of prostate cancer. *FASEB J.* 2020;34(4):4984–4996.

24. Clifford BK et al. Barriers and facilitators of exercise experienced by cancer survivors: a mixed methods systematic review. *Support Care Cancer.* 2018;26(3):685–700.

25. Pugh G et al. Trekstock RENEW: evaluation of a 12-week exercise referral programme for young adult cancer survivors delivered by a cancer charity. *Support Care Cancer.* 2020;28(12):5803–5812.

26. Gökler-Danışman I et al. Experience of grief by patients with cancer in relation to perceptions of illness: the mediating roles of identity centrality, stigma-induced discrimination, and hopefulness. *J Psychosoc Oncol.* 2017;35(6):776–796.

27. Faulkner A, Maguire P. *Talking to Cancer Patients and Their Relatives.* Oxford University Press; 1994.

28. Abbey G et al. A meta-analysis of prevalence rates and moderating factors for cancer-related post-traumatic stress disorder. *Psychoncology* 2015;24(4):371–381.

29. Riba MB et al. Distress management. *J Natl Compr Cancer Network.* 2019;17(10):1229.

30. O'Donnell E. The distress thermometer: a rapid and effective tool for the oncology social worker. *Int J Health Care Quality Assurance.* 2013;26(4):353–359.

31. Spitzer RL et al. 2006. A brief measure for assessing generalized anxiety disorder: the GAD-7. *Arch Intern Med.* 2006;22;166(10):1092–1097.

32. Kroenke K, Spitzer RL. The PHQ-9: 2002. A new depression diagnostic and severity measure. *Psychiatric Annals.* 2002;2:509–515.

33. Li M et al. Easier said than done: keys to successful implementation of the distress assessment and response tool (DART) program. *J Oncol Practice.* 2016;12(5): e513–e526.

34. Ownby KK. Use of the distress thermometer in clinical practice. *J Adv Pract Oncol.* 2019;10(2):175–179.

35. Johnston L et al. The implementation and impact of holistic needs assessments for people affected by cancer: a systematic review and thematic synthesis of the literature. *Eur J Cancer Care* 2019;28(3):e13087.

36. Chandwani KD et al. Cancer-related stress and complementary and alternative medicine: a review. *Evid Based Complement Alternat Med.* 2012:2012:979213.

37. Jarero I et al. Randomized controlled trial on the provision of the EMDR integrative group treatment protocol adapted for ongoing traumatic stress to female patients with cancer-related posttraumatic stress disorder symptoms. *J EMDR Pract Res.* 2018;12(3).

38. Xiao F et al. Effectiveness of psychological interventions on depression in patients after breast cancer surgery: a meta-analysis of randomized controlled trials. *Clin Breast Cancer.* 2017;17(3):171–179.

39. Howell D, et al. Management of cancer and health after the clinic visit: a call to action for self-management in cancer care. *J Nat Cancer Institute.* 2021;113(5):523–531.

40. Palmer Kelly E et al. The role of religion and spirituality in cancer care: an umbrella review of the literature. *Surg Oncol.* 2022;42:101389.

41. Elkins DN et al. Towards a humanistic-phenomenological spirituality: definition, description, and measurement. *J Humanist Psychology.* 1988;28(4):5–18.

42. Nolan S. Opening up the black box: how might we do spiritual assessment better? Oral presentation at CHCC Study Conference, 2019.

43. Sinclair S, Chochinov HM. The role of chaplains within oncology interdisciplinary teams. *Curr Opin Support Palliat Care.* 2012;6(2):259–268.

44. Yalom ID. Staring at the sun: overcoming the terror of death. *Humanist Psychol.* 2008;36(3–4):283–297.

45. Diet, Nutrition, Physical activity and cancer: a global perspective, third edition [internet], available at: https://www.wcrf.org/wp-content/uploads/2021/02/Summary-of-Third-Expert-Report-2018.pdf (accessed Mar 2023).

46. Cederholm T et al. Espen guidelines on definitions and terminology of clinical nutrition. *Clin Nutr.* 2017;36(1):49–64.

47. Fact sheets - malnutrition. World Health Organization. World Health Organization [internet], 2021, available at: https://www.who.int/news-room/fact-sheets/detail/malnutrition (accessed Mar 2023).

48. Muscaritoli M et al. 2012. Espen practical guideline: clinical nutrition in cancer. *Clin Nutr.* 2012;40(5):2898–2913.

49. Murphy JL et al. The provision of nutritional advice and care for cancer patients: a UK national survey of healthcare professionals. *Supportive Care in Cancer.* 2020;29(5):2435–2442.

50. Caccialanza R et al. Awareness and consideration of malnutrition among oncologists: insights from an exploratory survey. *Nutrition.* 2016;32(9):1028–1032.

51. Arends J et al. ESPEN guidelines on nutrition in cancer patients. *Clin Nutr.* 2017;36(1):11–48.

52. Alvarez-Hernandez J et al. Prevalence and costs of malnutrition in hospitalized patients; the PREDyCES Study. *Nutr Hosp.* 2012;27(4):1049–1059.

53. Molfino A et al. Current screening methods for the risk or presence of malnutrition in cancer patients. *Cancer Managers Res.* 2022;14:561–567.

54. Mendes NP et al. Nutritional screening tools used and validated for cancer patients: a systematic review. *Nutr Cancer.* 2019;71(6):898–907.

55. Jager-Wittenaar H. Assessing nutritional status in cancer. *Curr Opin Clin Nutr Metab Care.* 2017;20(5):322–329.

56. Nutritional Assessment [internet], BAPEN, available at (https://www.bapen.org.uk/education/nutrition-support/assessment-planning/nutritional-assessment/ (accessed Mar2023).

57. Cederholm T et al. GLIM criteria for the diagnosis of malnutrition – a consensus report from the global clinical nutrition community. *J Cachexia, Sarcopenia, Muscle.* 2019;10(1):207–217.

58. Ravasco P. Nutrition in cancer patients. *J Clin Med* 2019;8(8):1211.

59. Prado CM et al. Nutrition interventions to treat low muscle mass in cancer. *J Cachexia, Sarcopenia, Muscle.* 2020;11(2):366–380.

60. Centers for Disease Control, Cancer Care Settings and Smoking Cessation [internet], 2024, available at: https://www.cdc.gov/tobacco/hcp/patient-care-settings/cancer.html?CDC_AAref_Val=https://www.cdc.gov/tobacco/patient-care/care-settings/cancer/index.htm.

61. Cooley M et al. Smoking cessation interventions in cancer care: opportunities for oncology nurses and nurse scientists. *Annual Review Nurse Res.* 2009;27:243–272.

62. Project CURE [internet], available at: https://gmcancer.org.uk/the-cure-project/ (accessed Jan 2023).

63. Office for Health Improvement and Disparities, Nicotine vaping in England 2022 [internet], available at: https://www.gov.uk/government/publications/nicotine-vaping-in-england-2022-evidence-update/nicotine-vaping-in-england-2022-evidence-update-main-findings (accessed Jan 2023).

64. World Population Review, Smoking rates by country [internet], available at: https://worldpopulationreview.com/country-rankings/smoking-rates-by-country (accessed Jan 2023).

65. University of Plymouth, Very brief advice smoking cessation [internet], available at: https://www.plymouth.ac.uk/research/primarycare/global-health-research/very-brief-advice-smoking-cessation (accessed Jan 2023).

66. Macmillan Cancer Care, Cancer information and support [internet], available at: https://www.macmillan.org.uk/cancer-information-and-support/treatment/coping-with-treatment/giving-up-smoking (accessed Jan 2023).

67. Hartmann-Boyce J et al. Electronic cigarettes for smoking cessation. *Cochrane Database Syst Rev.* 2021;9(9).

68. Gallup. What percentage of Americans vape? [internet], 2022, available at: https://news.gallup.com/poll/267413/percentage-americans-vape.aspx (accessed Jan 2023).

69. Adriaens K et al. Effectiveness of the electronic cigarette: an eight-week Flemish study with six-month follow-up on smoking reduction, craving and experienced benefits and complaints. *Int J Environmental Public Health.* 2014;11(11):11220–11248.

Section IV

Special Populations

6

The Age Spectrum

6A

Older People and Frailty

Fabio Gomes and Martine Puts

Introduction

Most patients diagnosed with cancer around the world are older adults.[1] With the world population aging, the number of older adults diagnosed with cancer will rapidly increase in the next two decades. As patients age, their health and function can vary significantly, resulting in an increasingly heterogeneous population independent of chronological age.[2,3]

A challenge occurring frequently with increased age is frailty, which has been described by Ethun et al.[4] as "a complex, multidimensional, and cyclical state of diminished physiologic reserve that results in decreased resiliency and adaptive capacity and increased vulnerability to stressors" (Figure 6A.1). With increasing age, the prevalence of frailty increases, and several systematic reviews have consistently reported pooled frailty prevalence rates of 42–45% in older adults with cancer.[5–7] Alongside an increase in the frailty prevalence, older adults with cancer also have a higher prevalence of multimorbidity, with a complex interplay between frailty, chronic diseases, and disability (Figure 6A.2). Due to frailty, the risks of treatment may be higher compared to other populations owing to the lack of physical and psychological reserves to cope with the cancer and its treatments.

Frailty in older adults increases the risk for adverse outcomes such as functional decline, hospitalization, and early mortality and for patients receiving treatment for cancer it can increase the risk of post-operative complications, chemotherapy toxicity, and poorer prognosis.[4–7] Treatment benefits and risks also change due to the physiological aging processes, remaining life expectancy, and cancer and other health problems. This can lead to both over- and under-treatment[8] impacting cancer treatment outcomes and suboptimal use of scarce health care resources. This is particularly aggravated by a lack of evidence on how to best treat older adults with cancer as this population has been severely under-represented in clinical trials, particularly those with frailty,[9–12] racialized adults, and females.[13,14] Older adults, particularly those with frailty, are more likely to face ageism,[15] racism,[16–20] and (female patients) sexism[21] which can all interact and lead to poorer health care delivery and cancer outcomes.

DOI: 10.1201/9781003369912-13

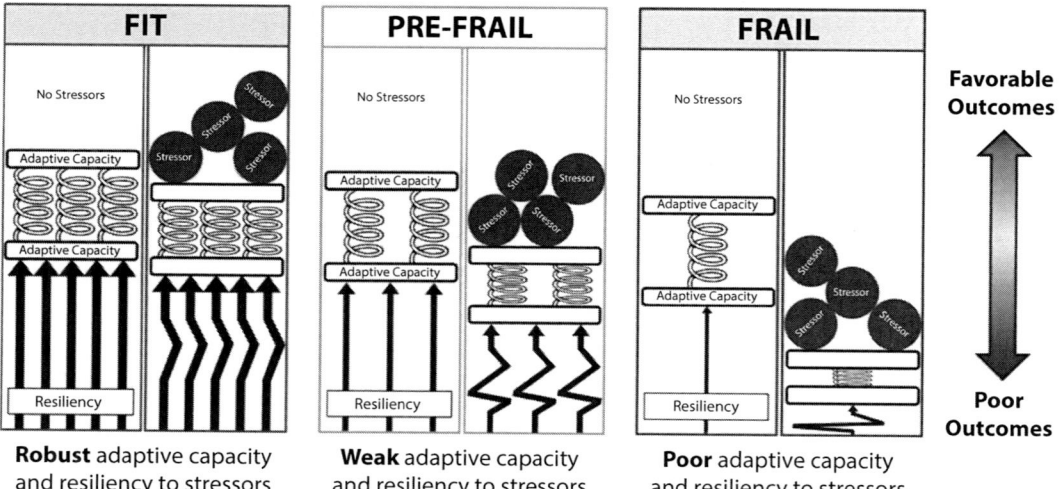

FIGURE 6A.1

A model for defining frailty. Fit patients have robust adaptive capacity and resiliency to stressors, which leads to more favourable outcomes. Prefrail patients have weakened adaptive capacity and resiliency to stressors, and frail patients have poor adaptive capacity and resiliency to stressors. Prefrail and frail patients are at greater risk of poor outcomes following surgery, chemotherapy, and radiotherapy. (Reproduced from ref 4 with permission.)

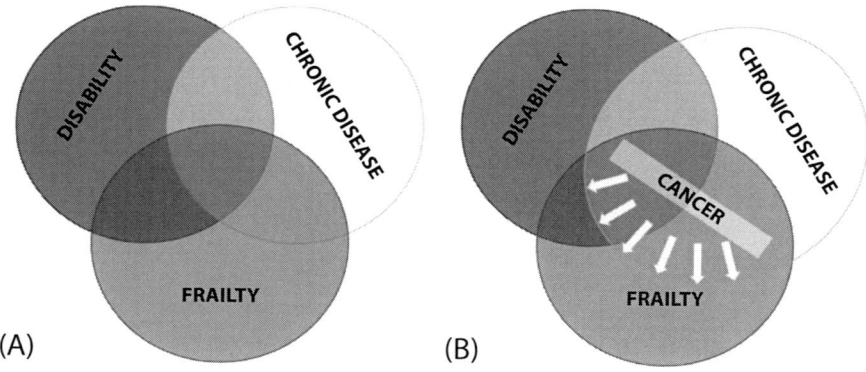

FIGURE 6A.2

The overlapping existence of frailty with disability and chronic disease (A). When chronic disease includes cancer, patients are at greater risk of having disability and frailty (B). (By courtesy of Drs Cecilia G. Ethun and Viraj A. Master.)

The decision-making process for these older patients with frailty is, therefore, far more complex. The risk of over-treatment must be considered, which is often due to an under-appreciation of the patient's frailty status. But the risk of under-treatment is also commonly observed, as ageism in oncology may lead to older adults being denied appropriate cancer care because they are considered "too old or too frail" to benefit from cancer treatments. Whilst it would be unreasonable to expect the treatment options and cancer outcomes for older patients with frailty to be the same as in younger and fit patients, there is high-level evidence supporting the need for improvement in care for older patients, aligned with their goals of care and values.

In this chapter we will review critical issues in the care for older adults with cancer and provide guidance on how to measure the level of frailty in an older adult and what can be done to ensure patient-centred high-quality cancer care.

Critical Issues in the Management of Older People Affected by Cancer

Older adults are more likely to experience both frailty and cancer.[22] Older adults account for about half of cancer cases worldwide,[23] and about 40% of these have some degree of frailty.[5–7] These patients are more vulnerable to functional impairments, and more likely to require input from different health care specialists throughout their cancer journey. Therefore, this is not a problem of tomorrow, but today's reality in oncology practices worldwide, and services must future proof themselves to support a growing number of older patients with complex needs.

Early diagnosis of cancer is key to provide the best outcomes to patients, yet data on older patients with frailty is scarce. But in its absence, the role of frailty can be inferred using multimorbidity data instead as a surrogate, considering these are often linked. Several studies suggest that older patients with multimorbidity are more likely to be diagnosed with prostate and breast cancer earlier than their healthier counterparts, which is possibly because of an enhanced medical monitoring.[24,25] However, in those older patients with cognitive decline, reports show that they instead are more likely to be diagnosed at a later stage, and more likely to receive a non-invasive diagnosis.[26–28]

Once an older patient is diagnosed with cancer, depending on the tumour and its stage, a surgical option may be an option under consideration. However, frailty is a strong positive predictor for post-operative complications,[29–33] and several scoring systems have been developed specifically for this purpose incorporating frailty parameters.[34,35] Whilst surgery may not be the best option for most older patients with frailty, carefully selected and appropriately supported older patients with some vulnerabilities and mild frailty may tolerate surgical treatments and benefit from them.[36,37]

Non-surgical treatments, such as radiotherapy and the large range of systemic anti-cancer treatments like chemotherapy and immunotherapy, are much more widely used for this group of patients. Radiotherapy is often used for example when systemic anti-cancer treatments are considered high-risk, due to its generally milder toxicity profile in a palliative setting. For example, shorter courses of radiotherapy have been developed for frail patients diagnosed with glioblastoma multiforme.[38] Data on the correlation between frailty and radiotherapy toxicity/tolerance is conflicting, with most studies unable to find a clear correlation with frailty whilst a positive correlation was found with older age (particularly 85+).[39–43]

Chemotherapy toxicity has largely been associated with frailty and consequently it is widely recommended that older patients aged 65+ are assessed for frailty before starting treatments.[44–46]

A well-recognized tool to predict toxicity is the Cancer and Aging Research Group (CARG) tool[47] and the Chemotherapy Risk Assessment Scale for High-age patients (CRASH) tool.[48] This can be used to help shared decision-making discussions with patients. A landmark trial in this space was the GO2 phase 3 trial which evaluated the optimal dosing of oxaliplatin and capecitabine in older patients with frailty and gastro-oesophageal cancer who were deemed unfit for full-dose triplet chemotherapy.[49] The study found that the lowest dose level of 60% was non-inferior in terms of progression-free survival, and patients experienced less toxicity and had a better overall treatment utility (OTU). The OTU is an innovative composite endpoint with patient- and clinical-reported outcomes. A good OTU meant there was disease control, no significant toxicity, no significant drop in quality of life, and a positive patient valuation of the treatment. Frailty was an independent predictor of OTU outcomes.

This study highlights an important point – due to under-representation of older patients in most clinical trials for drug development, frail patients often face limited treatment options, and a modified regimen with lower toxicity risks may not compromise disease control and provide any benefit to patients.

A more recent development within the systemic anti-cancer treatment arena has been the expanding use of immunotherapy with checkpoint inhibitors. As these treatments manipulate the immune system, concerns were raised that since older patients are more likely to have a dysfunctional immune system they may face higher treatment risks than younger people.[50] This has not been confirmed and immunotherapy is now widely used in these patients and recognized for its usually milder toxicity profile in most cases than chemotherapy, therefore potentially a better fit for many older patients with frailty. The ELDERS study looked specifically at the safety of immunotherapy in older patients with frailty and a diagnosis of lung cancer or malignant melanoma.[51] The ELDERS study showed there was no increase in the incidence of high-grade toxicity for these patients compared with their younger and fitter counterparts; however the older patients had a higher admission rate during treatment, likely reflecting their complex health status and a reduced capacity to cope with side effects.

Due to the multidimensional nature of frailty, older patients with cancer should be supported by multidisciplinary teams, engaging different experts such as oncologists, geriatricians, nursing, clinical pharmacy, physiotherapy, occupational therapy, and dietetics. Older patients with cancer and frailty also benefit from supportive care strategies. Therefore, supportive oncology experts also have a key role with these patients, particularly in the management of cancer symptoms and toxicities of cancer therapy, providing supportive care measures that could help patients with frailty to complete the planned treatment. Some symptoms may be more common in older adults with cancer and frailty. Therefore, in addition to multidisciplinary care, a focus on unique toxicities and on caregiver support is essential.

The early provision of palliative care is well-recognized particularly for those patients with a poorer prognosis, improving quality of life and preserving function as much as possible. For patients whose cancer and frailty preclude active cancer therapy, the provision of palliative care to alleviate cancer symptom burden may be the best and primary treatment strategy.

Deploying Geriatric Assessments to Improve Cancer Outcomes in Older Adults

Comprehensive Geriatric Assessment (CGA) is the gold standard to identify geriatric syndromes and frailty, and it is a multidimensional, interdisciplinary, diagnostic process to identify care needs, plan care, and improve outcomes of older adults with frailty.[52,53]

CGA is recommended by key oncology societies such as the American Society of Clinical Oncology (ASCO)[44,45] and the International Society of Geriatric Oncology (SIOG)[46] to be implemented for older adults over 65 years old with cancer who are being considered for cancer treatment. By recognizing that common vulnerabilities or impairments in older patients are not routinely captured in oncology assessments, undergoing a CGA aids with the cancer treatment decision and it also allows impairments to be addressed through non-oncology specific interventions (before and/or during the cancer treatment).

Systematic reviews have shown that CGA can impact treatment decisions for about 30% of older adults, mostly by identifying that the older patient was 'frailer' than previously thought and thus reducing the intensity of treatment to avoid adverse effects.[54] However, the CGA also leads to non-oncological interventions to improve health and functional status issues identified in the CGA, with Hamaker et al. reporting non-oncological interventions for about 70% of patients.[54]

A CGA should include the high-priority aging-related domains: Physical (including falls) and cognitive function, emotional health, comorbid conditions, polypharmacy, nutrition, and social support. There is a wide range of different tools to aid in assessing each domain and there is no consensus on the best way to assess each domain, but it is key that each domain is assessed. The ASCO published in 2023 an update of its original 2018 guideline with a helpful practical guide on how to assess and cover each domain (Table 6A.1).[45]

Collectively, the different CGA domains are interdependent. The functional status of the patient is dependent on the different domains, whereby an increasing number of impairments or vulnerabilities within and across domains correlates with an increased risk of functional dependency. Therefore considering functional status as an outcome measure is

TABLE 6A.1

Practical Geriatric Assessment

Domain	Measure	Definition of Impairments
Physical function	– Falls in the last 6 months – Walking one block or climbing one flight of stairs – 4-meter gait speed	– ≥1 falls – Any limitation (a little or lot) – Time ≥4 seconds (or gait speed ≤1.0 m/s)
Functional status	– OARS ADL – OARS IADL	– Any IADL items with some help or unable – Any ADL items with some help or unable
Nutrition	– Involuntary weight loss during the past 3 months	– Weight loss >3 kg (6.6 lbs)
Social support	– MOS social support tool	– Any instrumental or emotional item answered with "none; a little; some of the time"
Psychological	– GDS 5	– Score 2+
Comorbidity	– OARS comorbidity – Hearing and Vision	– 3+ conditions or any with great deal of interference – Fair/poor/deaf or blind
Cognitive function	– Mini-Cog	– Score 0–2
Risk of chemotherapy toxicity	– CARG toxicity tool	– Score 10–23 high risk

Note: Adapted from[45].

ADL: basic activities of daily living (in/out of bed, dressing, bath/shower); CARG: Cancer and Aging Research Group; GDS: Geriatric Depression Scale; IADL: Instrumental activities of daily living (walking, transportation, preparing meals, housework, managing medications, managing money); MOS: Medical Outcomes Survey; OARS: Older Americans Resources and Services.

key for older patients with cancer, and maintaining function, quality of life, and cognition are key considerations for older adults when considering cancer treatment.

Many screening tools have been developed to assess older people with the aim of better distinguishing those who are potentially fit.[4,55] The most widely recommended frailty screening tool in the field of geriatric oncology is the Geriatric-8 tool (G8)[56] followed by the Vulnerable Elder Survey 13 tool (VES-13).[57] The G8 was designed specifically for cancer patients aged 70+ and consists of 8 questions, with a score of 14 or lower (out of 17) meaning a positive screen. The VES-13 was validated in cancer patients aged 65+, consisting of 13 items and a positive screening meaning a score of 3 or above (out of 13). These screening tools take on average 5 minutes to apply and those who screen positive should then proceed to a CGA which may take about 60–90 minutes, depending on the complexity and number of vulnerabilities identified.

For years a key limiting factor to deploying CGA in oncology was the limited evidence that it would improve the clinical outcomes of older patients with cancer. But since 2020 several randomized clinical trials (RCTs) of CGA for older adults with cancer have been completed in different countries with different models and with different patient populations (Table 6A.2). Three of the RCTs focused on recruiting only older adults with frailty: GERICO, COACH, and GAP-70. The GERICO study used the G8 to identify older adults with frailty for inclusion in the RCT.[58] The COACH[59] and GAP-70[60] studies examined a CGA completed by the oncologist with a computer-generated list of recommendations to address the identified issues. Participants had advanced stage cancer in both studies and had to have at least one CGA domain impaired to be eligible for the study. All these RCTs showed significant benefits of the CGA in terms of improved quality of life, increased rates of treatment completion, reduced treatment toxicity, reduced falls, and higher number of medications stopped. The remaining five RCT summarized here (Table 6A.2) did not solely focus on older adults with frailty despite these representing the majority. With the exception of two RCT where no benefit was identified (5C study[61] and EGeSOR[62]) three other RCTs showed significant benefits from CGA in terms of reducing treatment toxicity,[63] improving functional status,[64] and improving quality of life.[65]

This growing number of RCTs has clearly showed the benefits in clinical outcomes of implementing CGA for older adults, particularly those with frailty, for whom cancer treatment is considered. This is particularly clear in term of toxicity, where a recent meta-analysis confirmed that the number of patients reporting treatment toxicity in the CGA groups was significantly lower compared with the usual care group (risk ratio 0.78 with a 95% confidence interval 0.70–0.86).[66]

The negative RCT EGeSOR deployed a standardized CGA which was delivered pre-treatment by a geriatrician with a follow-up for 24 months.[62] This implied failure of the chosen intervention model, suggesting that other models, such as co-management with oncologists and/or experienced practice nurses, could be useful in this setting. The 5C study[61] which also showed no significant impact of CGA on any study outcomes, showed that CGA conducted after the start of cancer treatment may be less effective in improving outcomes and that the conduct of a CGA should be completed prior to treatment selection. This aligns with a health economist evaluation modelling the cost-effectiveness of CGA, where the most cost-effective model was pre-chemotherapy with a nurse-led configuration.[67] So far, only the G-oncoCOACH study used a nurse-led CGA model.[65] Another key economic evaluation showed that CGA is more cost-effective for patients with cancer treated with a curative intent.[68]

Ultimately, different models of delivering a CGA can be effective in improving cancer treatment outcomes in different settings, ranging from oncologist-completed CGA to

TABLE 6A.2
Overview of the Pivotal RCTs of Geriatric Assessment for Older Adults with Cancer

RCT Name, Lead Author, and Year of Publication	N	Description of Population	Description of Intervention	Outcomes Summary
GERICO study, Lund 2021[58]	142	Median age was 75 and 43% were female. The study was conducted at 2 hospitals in Denmark.	A GA at baseline by a geriatrician with follow-up, compared to usual care.	Significantly more patients in the IG group completed scheduled chemotherapy compared to CG (45% vs. 28%). QoL significantly improved in IG compared with CG for the EORTC QLQ Elderly Subscales decreased burden of illness and improved mobility.
COACH study, Mohile 2021[59]	541	Mean age was 77 and 49% were female. The study was conducted at 31 community oncology practices in the USA.	A GA at baseline by oncologist for all but only IG received a list of recommendations.	The intervention led to improved satisfaction with more communication about age-related issues.
GAP-70 study, Mohile 2021[60]	718	Mean age was 77 and 43% were female. The study was conducted at 40 community oncology practices in the USA.	A GA at baseline by oncologist for all but only IG received a list of recommendations.	The IG had significant less grade 3–5 treatment toxicity (51%) compared to the CG, also fewer falls (12% vs to 21%), and more medications discontinued.
GAIN study, Li 2021[63]	605	Median age was 71 and 59% were female. The study was conducted in a single centre in the USA.	A GA at baseline by multidisciplinary team with the results sent to the oncologist for the CG, but with team follow-up for the IG.	The IG had significantly less grade 3–5 treatment toxicity (50.5% versus 60.6% in the CG) and more Advanced Care Directives completed compared to CG (28.4% versus 13.3%).
Integerate, Soo 2022[64]	154	Mean age 76 and 43% were female. The study was conducted at 2 hospitals in Australia.	A GA at baseline by geriatrician with follow-up, compared to usual care.	Participants in the IG had significantly better ELFI scores than CG. The IG also had significantly fewer hospital admissions.
5C study, Puts 2023[61]	350	Mean age was 76 and 40% were female. The study was a multicentre study at 8 hospitals in Canada.	A GA at baseline by nurse and geriatrician with follow-up by nurse, compared to usual care.	No significant findings on any outcomes.

(Continued)

TABLE 6A.2 (CONTINUED)

Overview of the Pivotal RCTs of Geriatric Assessment for Older Adults with Cancer

RCT Name, Lead Author, and Year of Publication	N	Description of Population	Description of Intervention	Outcomes Summary
EGeSOR, Paillaud 2022[62]	499	Mean age 75 and 31% were female. The study was conducted at 13 hospitals in France. Only patients with H&N cancer.	A GA at baseline by geriatrician with a standardized geriatric intervention and follow-up for 2 years, compared to usual care.	No significant findings on any outcomes.
G-oncoCOACH study, Peeters 2023[65]	212	Mean age was 77 and 52% were female. The study was conducted at 2 Belgian academic hospitals.	A GA at baseline by nurse with recommendations to oncologist for everyone, but only IG received nurse-led implementation of recommendations.	After 6 months, the difference between CG and IG showed significantly higher scores for the EORTC QLQ C30 Global Health subscale of 12.8 points in favour of the IG.

CG = control group; EORTC QLQ C30 = European Organisation of Research and Treatment of Cancer Quality of Life Questionnaire Core 30 items; ELFI score = Elderly Function Index score; H&N = head and neck; IG = intervention group.

dedicated multidisciplinary teams. Thus, the model of CGA may be selected by each centre dependent on the resources available.

Despite the recent evidence of the benefits of CGA and recommendations to implement it, there has been a slow uptake in routine oncology care for various reasons, including lack of knowledge on how to conduct a CGA and its proven benefits, a perception that it is too time-consuming, and a lack of resources to deploy it.[69–71] Whilst the latest RCT evidence may provide the evidence supporting the implementation of CGA in routine care, clinical teams will need to review what works best in their setting and with the resources available to them. There are multiple professional organizations, some national and other international such as the SIOG, which deliver workshops and regular meetings to help address the lack of knowledge on how to use frailty screening tools and deploy CGA in different clinical practices.[72]

Conclusion

The prevalence of frailty in older patients with cancer is high and there is often a complex interplay between frailty, chronic disease, and disability. The decision-making about cancer treatments can be particularly challenging in older patients, particularly with frailty, due to scarce evidence and the high risk of under- or over-treatment. The need for more clinical trials designed for treatment development which are more representative of this growing population has never been so critical. However, since 2020, there have been several landmark clinical trials completed further supporting that CGA must be implemented in routine clinical care, considering the clear improvement in the clinical outcomes for the rapidly growing number of older patients with cancer. There are different models to deploy CGA as best suited to each clinical practice and the resources available. But deploying CGA, particularly before a cancer treatment is started, showed the greatest benefit in several clinical outcomes, by aiding the treatment decision-making and then supporting patients with non-oncology specific interventions during their treatments. Due to these recent developments in the field, the routine use of CGA in cancer patients is anticipated to expand across different countries. But expanding the evidence, alongside raising awareness, and providing dedicated training to the multidisciplinary team continue to be paramount.

Top Tips for Geriatric Assessment

- Pick tools that work in your setting (self-administered by patient, clinician-administered).
- Pick a screening tool that can be easily used by everyone.
- Before you assess, make sure there is a management plan for what you will do for an impairment in that GA domain (e.g., know when to refer to dietician).
- Consider collecting some information for the GA over the phone prior to the visit to shorten the visit for the patient.
- Make sure the area where the assessment takes place is quiet, and patients have their assistive devices available for the tests (e.g., hearing aids, glasses, cane/walker) so that the assessment is a true assessment of their capabilities.

Pros and Cons: Geriatric Assessment

- There is clear evidence that using GA for older adults with cancer can significantly reduce treatment toxicity, and GA is recommended for all older adults.
- It provides an opportunity to develop a supportive care plan to avoid adverse effects of treatment.
- It takes time and trained staff to do these GAs.
- There needs to be a clear plan in place for what to do with impairments in the GA.

References

1. Pilleron S et al. International trends in cancer incidence in middle-aged and older adults in 44 countries. *J Geriatr Oncol*. 2022;3(3):346–55.
2. Nguyen QD et al. Health heterogeneity in older adults: exploration in the Canadian longitudinal study on aging. *J Am Geriatr Soc*. 2021;69(3):678–87.
3. Ferrucci L, Kuchel GA. Heterogeneity of aging: individual risk factors, mechanisms, patient priorities, and outcomes. *J Am Geriatr Soc*. 2021;69(3):610–2.
4. Ethun CG et al. Frailty and cancer: implications for oncology surgery, medical oncology, and radiation oncology. *CA Cancer J Clin*. 2017;67(5):362–77.

5. Komici K et al. Frailty in patients with lung cancer: a systematic review and meta-analysis. *Chest.* 2022;162(2):485–97.

6. Wang S et al. The prevalence of frailty among breast cancer patients: a systematic review and meta-analysis. *Support Care Cancer.* 2022;30(4):2993–3006.

7. Handforth C et al. The prevalence and outcomes of frailty in older cancer patients: a systematic review. *Ann Oncol.* 2015;26(6):1091–101.

8. DuMontier C et al. Defining undertreatment and overtreatment in older adults with cancer: a scoping literature review. *J Clin Oncol.* 2020;38(22):2558–69.

9. Kanapuru B et al. Older adults in hematologic malignancy trials: representation, barriers to participation and strategies for addressing underrepresentation. *Blood Rev.* 2020;43:100670.

10. Mishkin GE et al. Update on enrollment of older adults onto national cancer institute national clinical trials network trials. *J Natl Cancer Inst Monogr.* 2022;2022(60):111–16.

11. van Marum RJ. Underrepresentation of the elderly in clinical trials, time for action. *Br J Clin Pharmacol.* 2020;86(10):2014–6.

12. White MN et al. Advanced pancreatic cancer clinical trials: the continued underrepresentation of older patients. *J Geriatr Oncol.* 2019;10(4):540–6.

13. Dymanus KA et al. Assessment of gender representation in clinical trials leading to FDA approval for oncology therapeutics between 2014 and 2019: a systematic review-based cohort study. *Cancer.* 2021;127(17):3156–62.

14. Ladbury C et al. Age, racial, and ethnic disparities in reported clinical studies involving brachytherapy. *Brachytherapy.* 2022;21(1):33–42.

15. Haase K et al. The state of ageims in cancer care: a scoping review. *Supportive Care in Cancer.* 2021;29(1):S78–S9.

16. Hung MC et al. Racial/ethnicity disparities in invasive breast cancer among younger and older women: an analysis using multiple measures of population health. *Cancer Epidemiol.* 2016;45:112–8.

17. Jassal JS, Cramer JD. Explaining racial disparities in surgically treated head and neck cancer. *Laryngoscope.* 2021;131(5):1053–9.

18. Jiang S et al. Racial disparities and considerations for active surveillance of prostate cancer. *Transl Androl Urol.* 2018;7(2):214–20.

19. Kirtane K, Lee SJ. Racial and ethnic disparities in hematologic malignancies. *Blood.* 2017;130(15):1699–705.

20. Printz C. Racism and racial inequities in health care rise to the forefront: amid the country's national reckoning on race, experts are renewing their focus on systemic racism in the health care system. *Cancer.* 2020;126(18):4081–2.

21. Mendis S et al. Sex representation in clinical trials associated with FDA cancer drug approvals differs between solid and hematologic malignancies. *Oncologist.* 2021;26(2):107–14.

22. Smith BD et al. Future of cancer incidence in the United States: burdens upon an aging, changing nation. *J Clin Oncol.* 2009;27(17):2758–65.

23. Pilleron S et al. Global cancer incidence in older adults, 2012 and 2035: a population-based study. *Int J Cancer.* 2019;144(1):49–58.

24. Vaeth PA et al. Limiting comorbid conditions and breast cancer stage at diagnosis. *J Gerontol A Biol Sci Med Sci.* 2000;55(10):M593–600.

25. Raval AD et al. Association between types of chronic conditions and cancer stage at diagnosis among elderly medicare beneficiaries with prostate cancer. *Popul Health Manag.* 2016;19(6):445–53.

26. Legg JS et al. Are women with self-reported cognitive limitations at risk for underutilization of mammography? *J Health Care Poor Underserved.* 2004;15(4):688–702.

27. Gorin SS et al. Treatment for breast cancer in patients with Alzheimer's disease. *J Am Geriatrics Soc.* 2005;53(11):1897–904.

28. Gupta SK, Lamont EB. Patterns of presentation, diagnosis, and treatment in older patients with colon cancer and comorbid dementia. *J Am Geriatrics Soc.* 2004;52(10):1681–7.

29. Makary MA et al. Frailty as a predictor of surgical outcomes in older patients. *J Am Coll Surg.* 2010;210(6):901–8.
30. Revenig LM et al. Too frail for surgery? Initial results of a large multidisciplinary prospective study examining preoperative variables predictive of poor surgical outcomes. *J Am Coll Surg.* 2013;217(4):665–70.e1.
31. Kristjansson SR et al. Comprehensive geriatric assessment can predict complications in elderly patients after elective surgery for colorectal cancer: a prospective observational cohort study. *Criti Rev Oncol Hematol.* 2010;76(3):208–17.
32. Clough-Gorr KM et al. Examining five- and ten-year survival in older women with breast cancer using cancer-specific geriatric assessment. *Eur J Cancer.* 2012;48(6):805–12.
33. Audisio RA et al. Shall we operate? Preoperative assessment in elderly cancer patients (PACE) can help. A SIOG surgical task force prospective study. *Criti Rev Oncol Hematol.* 2008;65(2):156–63.
34. Huisman MG et al. Screening for predictors of adverse outcome in onco-geriatric surgical patients: a multicenter prospective cohort study. *Eur J Surg Oncol.* 2015;41(7):844–51.
35. Shahrokni A et al. Development and evaluation of a new frailty index for older surgical patients with cancer. *JAMA Network Open.* 2019;2(5):e193545.
36. Montroni I et al. GOSAFE – Geriatric oncology surgical assessment and functional recovery after surgery: early analysis on 977 patients. *J Geriatr Oncol.* 2020;11(2):244–55.
37. Montroni I et al. Quality of life in older adults after major cancer surgery: the GOSAFE international study. *JNCI.* 2022;114(7):969–78.
38. Ghosh S et al. Improved cost-effectiveness of short-course radiotherapy in elderly and/or frail patients with glioblastoma. *Radiother Oncol.* 2018;127(1):114–20.
39. Szumacher E et al. Use of comprehensive geriatric assessment and geriatric screening for older adults in the radiation oncology setting: a systematic review. *Clin Oncol.* 2018;30(9):578–88.
40. Middelburg JG et al. Timed get up and go test and geriatric 8 scores and the association with (Chemo-)radiation therapy noncompliance and acute toxicity in elderly cancer patients. *Int J Radiation Oncol Biol Physics.* 2017;98(4):843–9.
41. Spyropoulou D et al. Completion of radiotherapy is associated with the Vulnerable Elders Survey-13 score in elderly patients with cancer. *J Geriatr Oncol.* 2014;5(1):20–5.
42. Keenan LG et al. Assessment of older patients with cancer: Edmonton Frail Scale (EFS) as a predictor of adverse outcomes in older patients undergoing radiotherapy. *J Geriatr Oncol.* 2017;8(3):206–10.
43. VanderWalde NA et al. Geriatric assessment as a predictor of tolerance, quality of life, and outcomes in older patients with head and neck cancers and lung cancers receiving radiation therapy. *Int J Radiation Oncol Biol Physics.* 2017;98(4):850–7.
44. Mohile SG et al. Practical assessment and management of vulnerabilities in older patients receiving chemotherapy: ASCO guideline for geriatric oncology summary. *J Oncol Pract.* 2018;14(7):442–6.
45. Dale W et al. Practical assessment and management of vulnerabilities in older patients receiving systemic cancer therapy: ASCO guideline update. *J Clin Oncol.* 2023;41(26):4293–312.
46. Wildiers H et al. International society of geriatric oncology consensus on geriatric assessment in older patients with cancer. *J Clin Oncol.* 2014;32(24):2595–603.
47. Hurria A et al. Validation of a prediction tool for chemotherapy toxicity in older adults with cancer. *J Clin Oncol.* 2016;34(20):2366–71.
48. Extermann M et al. Predicting the risk of chemotherapy toxicity in older patients: the chemotherapy risk assessment scale for high-age patients (CRASH) score. *Cancer.* 2012;118(13):3377–86.
49. Hall PS et al. Efficacy of reduced-intensity chemotherapy with oxaliplatin and capecitabine on quality of life and cancer control among older and frail patients with advanced gastroesophageal cancer: the GO2 phase 3 randomized clinical trial. *JAMA Oncol.* 2021;7(6):869–77.
50. Presley CJ et al. Immunotherapy in older adults with cancer. *J Clin Oncol.* 2021;39(19):2115–27.
51. Gomes F et al. A prospective cohort study on the safety of checkpoint inhibitors in older cancer patients – the ELDERS study. *ESMO Open.* 2021;6(1):100042.

52. Rubenstein LZ. Joseph T. Freeman award lecture: comprehensive geriatric assessment: from miracle to reality. *J Gerontol A Biol Sci Med Sci.* 2004;59(5):473–7.
53. Rubenstein LZ et al. Impacts of geriatric evaluation and management programs on defined outcomes: overview of the evidence. *J Am Geriatr Soc.* 1991;39(9 Pt 2):8S–16S; discussion 7S–8S.
54. Hamaker M et al. Geriatric assessment in the management of older patients with cancer - A systematic review (update). *J Geriatr Oncol.* 2022;13(6):761–77.
55. Baitar A et al. Implementation of geriatric assessment-based recommendations in older patients with cancer: a multicentre prospective study. *J Geriatr Oncol.* 2015;6(5):401–10.
56. Soubeyran P et al. Screening for vulnerability in older cancer patients: the ONCODAGE prospective multicenter cohort study. *PLoS One.* 2014;9(12):e115060.
57. Saliba D et al. The vulnerable elders survey: a tool for identifying vulnerable older people in the community. *J Am Geriatr Soc.* 2001;49(12):1691–9.
58. Lund CM et al. The effect of geriatric intervention in frail older patients receiving chemotherapy for colorectal cancer: a randomised trial (GERICO). *Br J Cancer.* 2021;124(12):1949–58.
59. Mohile SG et al. Communication with older patients with cancer using geriatric assessment: a cluster-randomized clinical trial from the national cancer institute community oncology research program. *JAMA Oncol.* 2020;6(2):196–204.
60. Mohile SG et al. Evaluation of geriatric assessment and management on the toxic effects of cancer treatment (GAP70+): a cluster-randomised study. *Lancet.* 2021;398(10314):1894–904.
61. Puts M et al. Impact of geriatric assessment and management on quality of life, unplanned hospitalizations, toxicity, and survival for older adults with cancer: the randomized 5C trial. *J Clin Oncol.* 2023;41(4):847–58.
62. Paillaud E et al. Effectiveness of geriatric assessment-driven interventions on survival and functional and nutritional status in older patients with head and neck cancer: a randomized controlled trial (EGeSOR). *Cancers.* 2022;14(13).
63. Li D et al. Geriatric assessment-driven intervention (GAIN) on chemotherapy-related toxic effects in older adults with cancer: a randomized clinical trial. *JAMA Oncol.* 2021;7(11):e214158.
64. Soo WK et al. Integrated geriatric assessment and treatment effectiveness (INTEGERATE) in older people with cancer starting systemic anticancer treatment in Australia: a multicentre, open-label, randomised controlled trial. *Lancet Healthy Longev.* 2022;3(9):e617–e27.
65. Peeters L et al. A multicenter randomized controlled trial (RCT) for the effectiveness of comprehensive geriatric assessment (CGA) with extensive patient coaching on quality of life (QoL) in older patients with solid tumors receiving systemic therapy: G-oncoCOACH study. *J Clin Oncol.* 2023;41(16_suppl):12000.
66. Anwar MR et al. Effectiveness of geriatric assessment and management in older cancer patients: a systematic review and meta-analysis. *JNCI.* 2023;115(12):1483–96.
67. McKenzie GAG et al. Geriatric assessment prior to cancer treatment: a health economic evaluation. *J Geriatr Oncol.* 2023;14(6):101504.
68. Sahakyan Y et al. Cost-utility analysis of geriatric assessment and management in older adults with cancer: economic evaluation within 5c trial. *J Clin Oncol.* 2023;42(1):59–69.
69. Dale W. Why is geriatric assessment so infrequently used in oncology practices? the ongoing issue of nonadherence to this standard of care for older adults with cancer. *JCO Oncol Pract.* 2022;18(7):475–7.
70. Dale W et al. How is geriatric assessment used in clinical practice for older adults with cancer? A survey of cancer providers by the American society of clinical oncology. *JCO Oncol Pract.* 2020:Op2000442.
71. McKenzie GAG et al. Implementation of geriatric assessment in oncology settings: a systematic realist review. *J Geriatr Oncol.* 2021;12(1):22–33.
72. Arora SP, Puts M. Lessons learned from organizing international society of geriatric oncology (SIOG) geriatric assessment workshops. *J Geriatr Oncol.* 2023;14(5):101528.

6B

Teenagers and Young Adults

Hanna Simpson and Bob Philips

Supportive oncology in teenagers and young adults (TYA) is, like many aspects of working with adolescence and emerging adulthood, both unremarkable and unique.

Amongst TYA professionals, there has always been a recognition that their patient needs during cancer treatment are full of competing developmental demands, challenges to treatment delivery, and the management of complex side effects and consequences of treatment.

Understanding the needs of this patient population requires enhanced knowledge and an understanding of the development of teenagers into adulthood.

Epidemiology of Cancer in Teenagers and Young Adults (Including Haematological)

Whilst individual malignancies in children and young people are rare, "cancer" as a whole is not a rare event in childhood or young adulthood. One in 600 children (under 16) will have experience of a malignancy – four times as common as childhood diabetes or cystic fibrosis. An average high school will have two pupils who have, or have had, cancer or would have been at that school if they had survived. Long-term survival proportions, living into adulthood and beyond, currently sit around 85%.[1]

Cancer remains the third leading cause of death in younger patients aged between 13 and 24.[2] Whilst this age range generates approximately only 1% of new cancer diagnoses each year, the overall impact on individual patients and their families is significant. Each year in the UK, 2000–2500 young people receive a diagnosis of cancer.[1] The gender distribution of cancer is roughly equal; around 1 in every 360 young males and 1 in every 380 in young females, with minimal variation by race or ethnicity.[1]

The most common diagnoses in TYA patients include:

- Leukaemia
- Lymphoma
- Brain tumours
- Germ cell tumours (males)/malignant melanoma (females)
- Carcinomas

DOI: 10.1201/9781003369912-14

Treatment outcomes and experiences for cancer across all ages continue to improve, but the impact of this is seen least within the TYA population.[3] Compared with the cancer outcomes for children, young patients fare worse (adjusted odds ratio for mortality 1.49).[4] This is seen within the same diagnoses; for example, in osteosarcoma the reported survival rates for those aged under 15 are 75%, with those 15–39 only 65%.[5] Why?

This may be due to an array of reasons but includes more difficult diagnostic pathways,[4] subtly different biology within the diseases,[6] less tolerated treatment regimes,[7] and poorer recruitment to clinical trials, even when access to those trials is equivalent.[8] Added to this, young patients have more challenging late consequences of treatment for those who survive.[9]

Management of Cancer in Teenagers and Young Adults

Broad approaches to treatment in a TYA population will be the same as with adults, with the common treatment modalities of surgery, radiotherapy, and chemotherapy regularly utilized. A diagnosis of cancer affects every relationship within the patient's circle, and a balanced and negotiated approach to care is required, recognizing that there is no universally right way to behave and no right or wrong way for the patient to feel.

'Age-appropriate' care is the usual way of describing this approach and includes considering how all these elements are delivered in a cognitively and emotionally appropriate way, within an environment which does not alienate the patient.[10]

Younger patients are often supported by parents, siblings, friends, a significant other, and perhaps their own children. They often feel they have to balance being the person they were pre-cancer and the person who they feel they become when having treatment. A diagnosis of cancer may generate a range of complex emotions that may be difficult for young people and their families to process. Being reassured that their response is 'normal' is a powerful message to hear from professionals at this time. Similarly, when a child is diagnosed with cancer (irrespective of their age) the parents might think: 'did I miss something?', 'is it my fault?', or 'could it be hereditary?'

How might these responses be best managed? For those involved in delivering care, it is important to learn about the family, their dynamics, and the approach they will take to providing care and support. It is often the family who provide the largest amount of care and parents will look to the professional team providing care to guide them, reassure them, and recognize when they need support.

Some young patients regress in their behaviour and require significantly more care and help than prior to their cancer diagnosis. They may need parents to help with washing, medicine management, attending appointments, and understanding what is happening to them. Often parents are unsure if they are providing enough support, too much or too little. As with patients of all ages, each individual is different, and each family comes with its own nuances for care and support which must be navigated through the journey of treatment and beyond.

Sibling Perspective and Experiences

The siblings of a young person with cancer can often feel the experience in a hidden way compared to other members of the family. They are often supported by extended family members as the focus may be on the person with cancer and no longer on them. This can be difficult if they are younger and usually have a higher need for parental support.

Ensuring that the school, college, university, or workplace is aware that they have a sibling of a young person undergoing treatment for cancer also helps build the network of support around the sibling. When the patient is in hospital it can be exceptionally difficult for the siblings who may be used to seeing their sibling at home (and looking well) and seeing them in hospital can make the stark reality of their cancer diagnosis undeniable.

Professionals should consider utilizing video calls and frequent visits to the hospital to ensure siblings feel part of the caring journey and maintain the relationships and bonds with their family.

Intimate Relationships, Sex, and Sexuality

Teenagers and young people diagnosed with cancer may have a partner or significant other who will be part of their support network. The role they have within the relationship may change as they become more focused on caring for their partner and supporting them through their treatment.

Whilst cancer can bring a relationship closer together, it may also highlight issues within the relationship which existed prior to the diagnosis. Sexual intercourse and intimate acts within the relationship may also change or not be possible due to the diagnosis or treatment and this can have a huge effect on the relationship between the young patient and their partner. Support around changes in relationships, sexual advice, and – separate but linked – support and advice related to fertility in the short and long term are also aspects of care which need to be explored and considered.

Young patients are more likely to express a queer sexuality or diverse gender identity than adults, with recent survey work showing 20% teenagers (without cancer) endorsing an LGBTQ+ aspect to their lives.[11] They may also be in a period of growing understanding, with complexities around "coming out" to their family and friends. As with queer adults affected by cancer, understanding how professionals should approach these issues through an intersectional lens is discussed in Chapter 7.

Children and Blended Families

Although current figures for how many young patients are presenting with children of their own is not routinely collected, some teenagers and young adults may already have children or a blended family. Consideration for the care and support needed should include consideration of children of various ages.[12] Children can often also take a caring role and need specific support themselves.

Education services and the wider support network for the family should be aware of the diagnosis and care plan. For young parents affected by cancer this is often a significant area of concern as they are anxious about their access to support, potential financial concerns, potential outcome of the treatment, and if they will survive.

Encouraging access to support services including charitable networks and local provisions for support is imperative. Young patients who are parents often feel they need to be everything and more all whilst having treatment; the professional team around them have a duty of care for their patient but also their family and their needs.

Peer Support

Peers are important to young patients. Sometimes they may feel their peer groups are more important than their family. Maintaining relationships and engagement with friends is a key component around engagement and compliance with treatment and support throughout the treatment trajectory. Peer support from both friends prior to the cancer diagnosis and the friends they make subsequently is often the main area of normality during treatment, providing both a distraction from treatment and the support that comes from friendships outside of the family environment.

Supporting opportunities to maintain friendships both within and outside of the hospital is key for both the young patient and their family, although they may look to the treating team for reassurance that this is encouraged and safe from an infection focus. Many teams have exceptional Youth Support Coordinators who work tirelessly to provide opportunities for peer interaction and normalizing of the changes to existing peer relationships. Youth Coordinators typically are responsible for developing programmes of activities that include recreation, community services and volunteering, fundraising, safeguarding, and input in MDTs.

Interventions, and the way we implement them, do vary when working with children, young people, teenagers, young adults, and their families.

Photobiomodulation

Photobiomodulation is the application of a particular wavelength of light to prevent or treat oral mucositis and can be particularly challenging in this age group; some of the devices are built for an adult mouth, making them difficult for younger children and some smaller teenagers to use.

Many teenagers have a reluctance to be awake during an in-patient stay; part of this is a natural change in the circadian cycles through adolescence which conflicts with the rigid timetables of institutions,[13] the lethargy and exhaustion of cancer therapies, or the use of somnolence-inducing anti-emetics (see below) which are favoured by some young patients.

In this setting, an approach to treatment which demands attendance at a timed clinic slot – especially a morning one – could fail. Implementation programmes which empower ward staff within inpatients units to deliver the therapy at a time suitable for the patient, and collaborative approaches with children as young as 5, such as holding the devices to give themselves therapy, can be employed. Preparing information designed and featuring young people along with 'play' units (mock devices which can be experienced without any possibility of harm or benefit) can also reduce the reluctance to cooperate with novel treatment programmes.

Nausea and Vomiting

The pharmacological management of nausea and vomiting follows similar patterns as in older cancer patients, but the menu of medications varies across age ranges, and the delineation of the risk of nausea/vomiting is far less well described.[14] Some of the challenges may appear obvious: For medications, dosing and formulation have been less well developed and studied for smaller and younger patients.[15] Other changes are more subtle: Multi-day regimens are the rule, rather than the exception; for many young patients, feeling drowsy through the hospital stay is a positive, and some actively enjoy some of the dissociative experiences associated with some of the antiemetics.

Pain

Pain management faces similar challenges and is associated with patients expressing greater sadness and worry. Some practitioners have strong concerns about the possibilities of opiate addiction and misuse, leading to under-treatment of painful episodes and a negative impact upon their quality of life.

Whilst systematic studies of the rates of opiate addiction for TYAs are limited, where research has been attempted the vast majority (around 90%) of young patients using opiates do so without any form of problematic use. An approach which assesses generic markers of risk, such as prior drug/alcohol misuse, multiple prescriptions, varied sources of opiate prescriptions, and focusing upon the painkiller over and above any other element of the consultation should be used to guide management.[16] The management of opioids for all patients in a supportive oncology setting is discussed in Chapter 3B.

There is a significant challenge around compliance, with many younger patients forgetting to take their analgesics consistently. Disciplined self-medication can be problematic for young patients where life has perhaps been less routine and regimented than adults. Creative approaches to reminders, longer-acting formulations, and non-standard timings can be more effective.

Do younger patients have the experience to understand how to engage with pain support effectively? Do they recognize that their feelings take time, support, and guidance to manage? With this in mind, should professionals be encouraged therefore to think 'outside the box'? One option might be to consider the potential for enhancing pharmacological measures through integrative and technological innovation including virtual reality and games.[17] Similarly, there may also be opportunities for the application of artificial intelligence (AI) in this area. The impact of AI on service development is discussed in Chapter 9.

Fever in Neutropenia

The management of neutropenic sepsis in adults is discussed in detail in Chapter 2, but with the greater intensity of therapies delivered to younger people affected by cancer, neutropenic sepsis is an even more common event in this cohort.

In children, 80% of those undergoing SACT will experience "febrile neutropenia", and the median is two episodes per year. International guidelines have been developed for the younger (<18) groups, concentrating on prompt recognition, risk-stratification, and appropriately weighted treatment.[18] Minimal hospitalization methods, with early discontinuation of antimicrobial therapies, have been effectively delivered in the UK.[19]

Work has shown the 'upscaling' of children's stratification schema, and the 'de-aging' of standard adult criteria, do not work as well to accurately stratify the risk of poor outcome in TYA patients.[7,20] Add to this the reluctance sometimes to disclose fever, or attend for assessment, and the management of potential life-threatening infection is spiced with the need for excellent TYA-facing staff to understand and educate patients and families.

Complementary Therapies

Nonpharmacological support mechanisms have a significant role in the supportive care needs of younger patients with complementary therapies, physical activity, and occupational therapy of particular importance.

The effectiveness of complementary therapy and the value of therapeutic touch for young patients is recognized across the whole of the cancer continuum. However, touch is often perceived negatively by young patients during the treatment phase, and it may take time for professionals to reintroduce touch therapy interventions that are acceptable once treatment has finished.

With more young patients becoming connected with ideas and practices in this space, perhaps through promotion on social media, through peer groups, or in educational settings, there is an opportunity for professionals to help patients develop self-management skills which will last through their treatment trajectory and into adulthood. Some teenage and young adult cancer charities have prioritized focusing on holistic wellbeing to help with managing symptoms and provide support for families. Professional teams should be encouraged to place this high on the supportive care agenda for this group of patients.

Physical Therapies

Physical therapy and prehab/rehab are often approached with trepidation as many young patients feel they have no energy or resilience to engage with this important part of their cancer treatment.[21] With cancer charities and the NHS placing ever increasing value on the benefits of physical activity in supportive care, it is imperative that a range of options to support exercise and activity are available for young patients.

Occupational therapy provides a range of interventions that focus on both the physical wellbeing of patients and their psychological and emotional needs and may be an important intervention to support a patient returning to education or the workplace, or independent living.

Other interventions include sleep therapy and talking therapies such as counselling. Deploying these interventions can be particularly helpful when considering the management of some of the top survivorship concerns including fatigue, anxiety around cancer coming back, and body image.

Despite advances in front-line cancer treatment, patients may be managing ongoing side effects for a considerable period after treatment has finished or encountering unexpected late consequences of treatment. Supportive oncology teams must consider the future and provide appropriate care which may resonate across a whole lifetime, both for the patient and their family.

References

1. Welham C, et al. Children, teenagers and young adults UK cancer statistics report 2021. Report on behalf of the National Cancer Registration and Analysis Service for England (Public Health England), the Northern Ireland Cancer Registry, the Scottish Cancer Registry (part of Public Health Scotland), and the Welsh Cancer Intelligence and Surveillance Unit (part of Public Health Wales) [internet], available from: http://ncin.org.uk/view?rid=4272.

2. Office for National Statistics. Mortality statistics by age, sex, and cause of death [internet], available from: https://www.ons.gov.uk/peoplepopulationandcommunity/birthsdeathsandmarriages/deaths/datasets/deathsregisteredinenglandandwales2021refreshedpopulations.

3. KeeganTH et al. Comparison of cancer survival trends in the United States of adolescents and young adults with those in children and older adults. *Cancer* 2016;122(7), 1009–1016.

4. Li M et al. Cancer profiles, times to treatment, and survival for adolescents and young adults: comparisons with children and older adults in New South Wales, Australia. *J Adolesc Young Adult Oncol* 2022;11(5), 443–450.

5. Alken S et al. Survival of childhood and adolescent/young adult (AYA) cancer patients in Ireland during 1994-2013: comparisons by age. *Irish J Med Sci* 2020;189(4):1223–1236.

6. Murray MJ et al. The two most common histological subtypes of malignant germ cell tumour are distinguished by global microRNA profiles, associated with differential transcription factor expression. *Mol Cancer* 2010;9:290.

7. Kirolos N et al. Does age play a role in fever and neutropenia events and complications: a comparison of adolescents versus younger children with cancer at a tertiary care paediatric hospital, a pilot project. *Cancer Rep* 2023;6(4):e1767.

8. Thomas SM et al. A prospective comparison of cancer clinical trial availability and enrollment among adolescents/young adults treated at an adult cancer hospital or affiliated children's hospital. *Cancer* 2018;124(20):4064–4071.

9. Chao C et al. Incidence, risk factors, and mortality associated with second malignant neoplasms among survivors of adolescent and young adult cancer. *JAMA Network Open* 2019;2(6):e195536.

10. Fern LA et al. The art of age-appropriate care: reflecting on a conceptual model of the cancer experience for teenagers and young adults. *Cancer Nurs* 2013;36(5):E27–E38.

11. Morris JN et al. The well-being of children impacted by a parent with cancer: an integrative review [published correction appears in Support Care Cancer. 2016;24(8):3677]. *Support Care Cancer.* 2016;24(7):3235-3251.

12. Gannon T et al. Knowing to ask and feeling safe to tell – understanding the influences of HCP-patient interactions in cancer care for LGBTQ+ children and young people. *Front Oncol.* 2022;12.

13. Crowley SJ et al. Sleep, circadian rhythms, and delayed phase in adolescence. *Sleep Med.* 2007;8(6):602–612.

14. Phillips RS et al. Antiemetic medication for prevention and treatment of chemotherapy-induced nausea and vomiting in childhood. *Cochrane Database Syst Rev.* 2016;2(2):CD007786.

15. Phillips B et al. Individual participant data validation of the PICNICC prediction model for febrile neutropenia. *Arch Dis Childhood.* 2019;105(5):439–445.

16. Pinkerton R, Hardy JR. Opioid addiction and misuse in adult and adolescent patients with cancer. *Int Med J.* 2017;47(6):632–636.

17. Jibb LA et al. Psychological and physical interventions for the management of cancer-related pain in paediatric and young adult patients: an integrative review. *Oncol Nurs Forum.* 2015;42(6):E339–E357.

18. Lehrnbecher T et al. Guideline for the management of fever and neutropenia in pediatric patients with cancer and hematopoietic cell transplantation recipients: 2023 update. *J Clin Oncol.* 2023;41(9):1774–1785.

19. Jackson TJ et al. Can I go home now? The safety and efficacy of a new UK paediatric febrile neutropenia protocol for risk-stratified early discharge on oral antibiotics. *Arch Dis Childhood.* 2022;108(3):192–197.

20. Phillips RS et al. Risk stratification in febrile neutropenic episodes in adolescent/young adult patients with cancer. *Eur J Cancer.* 2016;64:101–106.

21. Robinson PD et al. Management of fatigue in children and adolescents with cancer and in paediatric recipients of haemopoietic stem-cell transplants: a clinical practice guideline. *Lancet Child Adolesc Health.* 2018;2(5):371–378.

7

Intersectional Approaches to Supportive Oncology

Ben Heyworth, Charlotte Leach, and James Burtonwood

Introduction

Is good medicine a social process as well as a scientific or technical endeavour? Research that highlights the crucial role of good communication, interpersonal relationships, identity, geography, employment, and challenging stigmas in supporting good clinical outcomes would suggest so. Indeed, good health is multi-faceted and influenced by many factors usually referred to as the wider social determinants of health.

In all countries – whether low-, middle-, or high-income – there are wide disparities in the health status of different social groups, and whilst the biggest driver of health inequality globally is low socioeconomic status, oncology professionals across all care settings should routinely consider how individual characteristics intersect, exacerbating and compounding inequalities, and seek to address them.[1]

In supportive oncology, the intersectional impact of the wider social determinants of health can have a substantial impact on overall quality of life, patient experiences of care, and clinical outcomes. In this chapter, we will consider the importance of social and intersectional issues in the management of patients within a supportive oncology service.

Global Equality, Diversity, and Human Rights Legislation

There are wide disparities between different countries regarding the legal framework for the protection of minority "characteristics", often reflecting local cultural, religious, or political normality. An effective legal framework protecting individuals from discrimination can have a positive impact on health inequalities that may be present across a geography. Where countries have fewer protections for minority groups, there is a greater likelihood that these sections of the population will encounter barriers to effective healthcare, especially where targeted interventions are required that support the needs of a specific group.

In adopting the UN Agenda for Sustainable Development,[2] the UK has committed to meeting 17 sustainable development goals which include "reducing inequality", "gender equality", and "good health and wellbeing". Access to care and treatment should be based solely on clinical need, and the principle of equality sits at the very heart of the NHS constitution.[3]

DOI: 10.1201/9781003369912-15

However, inequalities in healthcare have persisted in the UK despite being recognized in both the Five Year Forward View[4] and the Long-Term Plan,[5] which both identified how a "one-size fits all" approach does not address the particular needs of individuals who may be culturally, racially, and sexually diverse.[6] Furthermore, patients are protected by the Equalities Act (2010)[7] which defines nine "protected" characteristics (race, age, gender, gender reassignment, marriage and civil partnership, pregnancy, faith, sexual orientation, and disability), making it illegal to discriminate against individuals who may identify with one or more category.

In the United States, constitutional change driven by the civil rights movement of the 1950s and 1960s has had a significant impact on legal, social, and political equality. The marginalization of African Americans spurred a social movement based mainly in churches and colleges of the South, where direct action including marches, boycotts, and civil disobedience, such as sit-ins, as well as voter education and voting drives, created a model for social activism that resonated around the world, including influencing the successful fight against apartheid in South Africa in the 1980s.

Other civil rights movements swiftly followed: For example, the US has made significant strides in LGBTQ+ rights over the years, coding an increasing number of LGBTQ+ rights into national law – for example, legalization around gay marriage and legalization around the adoption of children by same-sex couples. Undoubtably, the advancement of civil rights across the US has improved access to healthcare and reduced discrimination; however the biggest driver for health inequalities in the US is the reliance on private healthcare insurance, and those who have corporate-sponsored plans continue to have better access to healthcare than those who do not.

In China, despite deep-rooted Confucianism producing some of the strictest patriarchal social structures and state repression making the likelihood of social activism of the sort that drove change in the US unlikely, the State Council Information Office nevertheless published in 2005 a white paper entitled 'Gender Equality and Women's Development',[8] emphasizing the importance of women's rights, including participation in decision-making, access to education, and marital rights.[9] New rules aimed at clarifying gender equality laws and expanding women's workplace protections took effect in on 2019.[10] However, shifts towards religious freedom, LGBT rights, true gender equality, and other socially progressive causes continue to move forward at a glacial pace, if at all, under the conservative yet all-seeing eye of the Chinese Communist Party.

Most countries restrict rights to some minority groups, and it remains difficult for supra-national organizations such as the United Nations or the European Union to enforce standards in human rights. For minority groups facing discrimination, hope lies in governments feeling the pressure for social change from local activism and allyship, or external pressure from other governments. Meanwhile, the Universal Declaration of Human Rights, adopted by the United Nations in 1948, includes civil rights language but is not binding on member states.

Cultural Competency

Assuming the political, social, and legal landscapes safely allow providers to offer support to patients from minority groups seeking help in a particular geography, healthcare professionals should consider taking steps to equip themselves with the knowledge and skills required to deliver inclusive, holistic, person-centred care. This may entail further education and training, regular reflective practice, and practicing inclusive leadership skills. The terms "cultural competence" and "cultural humility" have become associated with good practice and workforce upskilling around equality, inclusion, and diversity, but what do these terms really mean? Is being "culturally competent" helpful in managing diverse patients and navigating health inequalities in supportive oncology settings?

Some commentators have suggested that the concept "cultural competence" shares two basic assumptions – that it is a necessary condition for working effectively with difference, and that it can be taught, learned, trained, and achieved.[11] Effective education and training – which might include acknowledging privilege, learning and deploying appropriate and inclusive language whilst remaining curious, whilst also recognizing the individual, being person-centric but avoiding stereotyping – would equip clinicians with a suitable skillset that we might describe as "cultural competence". Yet many professionals continue to express anxiety about inadvertently saying the wrong thing, using the wrong label, misgendering a patient, accidentally stereotyping, or otherwise causing offence.[12]

Missing from a "cultural competency" curriculum might be a discussion of wider issues that impact health inequality – experiences around restrictive laws or barriers, fears around deportation, tackling xenophobic and discriminatory attitudes amongst staff, and restricted access or lack of inclusion in health systems – and this is why it is important to take an intersectional perspective to tackling inequality that might go above and beyond this definition of "cultural competence".

It is through the evolution of language that communities construct safe spaces and inclusive environments. Consider the word "queer" – a word meaning strange, odd, or different, also once a derogatory term used to demonize, offend, and exclude LGBT people, now re-adopted to reflect a segmentation of the LGBT community and its allies that defines itself through queerness (or perhaps "questioning"), the word's power to offend considerably diminished.

The use of the terms black, Asian and minority ethnic (BAME) and black and minority ethnic (BME) provides another case in point. In March 2021, the Commission on Race and Ethnic Disparities (UK) recommended that these terms should not be used. It was felt that they emphasize certain ethnic minority groups (Asian and black) and exclude others (mixed, other, and white ethnic minority groups), masking disparities between different ethnic groups and creating misleading interpretations of data.

This was supported by research commissioned by the Race Disparity Unit (RDU), which found that people from ethnic minorities were 3 times more likely to agree than disagree that the term 'BAME' was unhelpful.

Language and labels used by minority groups are constantly changing, shifting, and developing. Professionals should remember to respectfully ask if they are unsure how an individual might identify, or which label they would use to describe themselves or their communities, if it is relevant to the immediate clinical presentation, diagnosis, or future care plan.

Understanding What We Mean by "Intersectionality" in Supportive Oncology

The term "intersectionality" was first described by American sociologist Kimberlé Crenshaw in 1989 and emerged from several closely related theories including black feminist, indigenous feminist, third-world feminist, queer, and postcolonial.[13] The theory encourages us to think less about individual factors such as sex, gender, biology, or race, and focus instead on the interactions between such factors, and subsequently highlighting that there are important differences within superficially homogenous population groups (e.g., women, migrants, visible minorities) that are often misunderstood or ignored.[14]

An intersectionality-informed health intervention should be able to describe more broadly the physical, psychological, emotional, economic, social, and vocational needs of a patient and to act accordingly. Intersectional theory underpins the widely understood notion of person-centred care and informs holistic care models including personalized care pathways and holistic needs assessments, and indeed any best practice in medicine that seeks to treat a patient, not just cure a disease.

A growing body of healthcare professionals are taking an intersectional approach to understanding why health inequalities occur.[15] An intersectional approach recognizes that an individual who identifies across multiple protected characteristics such as age, disability, or sexual orientation in combination with other determinants of health such as economic status and geography is more likely to encounter systems of oppression, including systemic discrimination. Intersectional approaches to healthcare are useful because they reduce the likelihood of overemphasizing cultural or ethnic differences in minority population groups, for example, through focusing on "cultural competencies" such as language or cultural barriers alone.

Intersectional approaches to practice within supportive oncology can provide a more nuanced understanding of patients and their circumstances. Interventions that target alcohol and tobacco use, unhealthy diets, and physical activity, but fail to consider the broader context that shapes these choices, behaviours, and specific realities of differently situated groups, are often ineffective.

Cancer and Homelessness through an Intersectional Lens

The term 'homelessness' encompasses a broad range of experiences, and the spectrum varies from transiently unstable living arrangements such as temporary accommodation with a friend (colloquially known as 'sofa-surfing'), emergency accommodation, those escaping abuse, persecution, or violence in a refuge, and those with a permanent lack of access to any shelter or amenities.[16]

Homelessness is an independent risk factor for all-cause mortality, often from preventable causes,[17-19] and a number of factors make patients who are (or have been) homeless more likely to develop cancer, present late, and have less effective treatment, including tobacco use, alcohol consumption, illicit drug use, significant sun-exposure, and viral infections; they are certainly a patient group for whom taking an intersectional view towards care planning and treatment would be preferable.

Supportive oncology teams need to be equipped to address a wide variety of potential safeguarding issues[20] and past trauma.[21] Poor experiences of the healthcare system or fear and mistrust of healthcare professionals/authorities may lead to disengagement from cancer services and in turn hinder a therapeutic relationship.[22] Many homeless patients are at risk of significant anxiety, distress, or reduced quality of life prior to cancer diagnosis;[23] these may become exacerbated after diagnosis.[24] There is, therefore, a need for the multidisciplinary, holistic approach which supportive oncology can provide yet valid concerns about equitable access remain; it is widely acknowledged that homeless patients are a 'difficult to reach' group.[25]

Patients and supportive oncology services may face important logistical barriers which must be overcome for effective and safe care. Liaison with social care services and local government is vital to provide prompt access to suitable accommodation and amenities. Many may find themselves accommodated in circumstances inadequate for their needs. Access issues, shared bathrooms, or lack of kitchen facilities may stymie some of the basic interventions needed for effective care. Many arrangements may be contingent on continued habitation and emergency admission or attendance for regular oncological therapy may risk forfeiture of accommodation.

Some temporary accommodation establishments may operate a strict no-drugs policy which poses difficulties in providing prescription opioids or benzodiazepines. Indeed, the possession of these medications in shared accommodation may make the patient vulnerable to theft or bullying. An added complication arises as opioid overdose is a leading cause of death in this population.[26] The use of illicit drugs may increase the risk of unintentional overdose. Concurrent methadone use may interact with other medications causing QT interval prolongation or increase the risk of opioid-toxicity. High doses of buprenorphine may interfere in pain relief through partial antagonism of opioids. Previous IV drug misuse may make IV access more challenging or extravasation more likely. Damage to blood vessels from recurrent injection may increase the risk of DVT or infection.

Other complicating factors include:

- Poor dentition which may limit the use of bisphosphonates.
- Poor oral hygiene increasing the risk of mucositis.
- Immunosuppression from conditions such as HIV.
- Poorly controlled diabetes or liver disease may make opportunistic infection more likely and difficult to manage.
- And communicable respiratory diseases such as TB or COVID may be more common in shared accommodation and can complicate treatment.

Financial difficulties may be exacerbated by the expense of travel to and from therapy appointments. Clinical teams should have access to advocates experienced in navigating the complexities of social support and financial benefits for the homeless. In some countries, care also needs to be taken to ensure patients are promptly exempted from prescription charges and not inadvertently asked to fund over-the-counter medications that would otherwise be provided for free.

Temporary addresses mean that communicating by letter is often impossible and lack of basic access to email or text messaging may make it challenging to arrange appointments, or indeed for the patient to seek help or advice. And homeless patients may face discrimination when trying to register for, or access, primary care services.

Supportive oncology teams must not ignore their vital advocacy role and ensure teams understand the issues and experiences of homeless patients to provide a flexible, pragmatic, trauma-informed approach.

Cancer and Sexual Orientation/Gender Identity Minorities (LGBT)

The LGBT community is not a homogenous group but encompasses a range of minority identities. Many people who describe themselves as members of the LGBT community use different labels to identify and express themselves. These include familiar terms such as 'gay', which describes any kind of same-sex attraction, 'lesbian', which has been adopted by some women who are attracted to other women, and 'bisexual', which relates to people who are attracted to men and women.

Why is it important to consider sexual orientation or gender identity in a supportive oncology setting? There may be specific and tailored interventions for LGBT people dealing with common issues – particularly with reference to sexual health and wellbeing. For example, recently developed guidance sets out an appropriate framework for safe sexual practice around giving and receiving anal sex for gay and bisexual men who have had treatment with radiotherapy to the pelvis for the first time.[27]

Healthcare professionals should not make assumptions on sexual orientation based on appearances and, in keeping with best practice in person-centred care, remain both respectful and sufficiently curious at a level appropriate to the clinical issue in question.

Gender minority groups are usually described under the umbrella term 'transgender', which applies to individuals whose gender expression does not match the gender they were assigned at birth and includes those who identify as non-binary, gender fluid, and no gender. This is distinct from biological sex, a term used to describe gender as assigned at birth and which relates specifically to physiognomy and anatomy, where gender identity encompasses the physical, psychological, social, and emotional experiences of identifying as a particular sex.[28]

Despite gender dysphoria no longer falling within the remit of mental illness in ICD-11, evidence of increased levels of mental distress amongst trans-identifying adults is substantial, usually attributed to societal responses to gender non-conformity.[29] There is a negative socio-political environment surrounding discussion of trans and non-binary identities. So called "gender critical" feminists raising concerns around women's safety in some "female-only" spaces (such as women's prisons) encounter counterclaims of transphobia and bigotry from the trans community and their allies who feel they are being unfairly stigmatized, given the weight of evidence that suggests most violence towards women in gendered spaces is perpetrated by cis-gender men not trans women.

This is leading to the constant threat of the erosion of legal rights – perhaps most starkly illustrated by some particularly draconian legislation introduced in 2022 across many of the southern states in the US, including restrictions to gender-affirming care, trans-affirmative education, participation and access to athletics, changes to birth certificates, and religious discrimination.[30] The impact of this on the mental health and wellbeing, and indeed personal safety, of trans people has been profoundly negative.

Are clinical professionals therefore finding this topic too hot to handle? Perhaps there is some reluctance to engage with the thorny issue of trans health from some clinicians, but in the UK, half a million people self-identify as trans, and this number is growing fast.

More younger people than ever are seeking medical help around gender identity, with referral rates to the UK's Gender Identity Development Service at the Tavistock Centre (Tavistock and Portman NHS Trust) in London rising from under 210 in 2011/12 to 3585 in 2021/22.[31] Perhaps the true impact on cancer services will only be felt as this section of the population ages.

Trans and non-binary people have a complex epidemiology, and there are significant cancer-related health inequalities. This group are more likely to be diagnosed late, more likely to encounter multiple and complex treatment problems, and more likely to have a poor experience of care. This situation is likely compounded by other factors including incomplete coding in clinical records, lack of recording of sex assigned at birth, and the absence of linked information for gender-affirming treatments and services should they be required. Most services are unlikely to deploy trans-inclusive gender identity and trans status demographic monitoring.

Cancer and Disability: d/Deaf, Sight Impairments, Intellectual Disabilities

Persons with disabilities encounter multiple health inequities. Disabilities may be physical, intellectual, and/or due to mental health conditions, and there is significant heterogeneity of the disability experience. Persons may have disabilities prior to their cancer and/or anti-cancer treatment or may experience disability because of cancer and/or anti-cancer treatment; for example, reduced arm movement resulting from breast cancer surgery.

Under the Equality Act (2010)[7] cancer is defined as a disability; however, not all persons with cancer consider themselves disabled.

In the United Kingdom, approximately 151,000 persons use British Sign Language (BSL).[32] The word Deaf refers to persons who were born Deaf or became Deaf pre-lingually, identify with Deaf culture and likely to use BSL; the word deaf refers to persons who have an acquired hearing impairment, and are more likely to use oral communication methods such as lip-reading.

Multiple inequalities and inequities exist in the access and delivery of culturally appropriate healthcare for Deaf persons including language barriers, lower levels of health knowledge compared to hearing persons, and cultural differences about healthcare. The Deaf community represent a heterogeneous population with different preferred communication methods. For many Deaf persons, English is a second language, and accessing healthcare information in their preferred language of BSL is frequently challenging. BSL is not a signed version of English, meaning that providing healthcare information in written English is often inadequate in meeting the needs of Deaf persons.

Supportive oncology teams must bear in mind that there is likely to be a difference between those persons who were d/Deaf prior to cancer diagnosis or anti-cancer treatment, and those persons who are deaf due to cancer or anti-cancer treatment. Deaf people often consider their deafness to be an integral aspect of their identity (called "Deaf identity"), rather than considering their Deafness as a disability or medical condition. Both Deaf culture and Deaf identity are likely to impact on a Deaf person's perspective and interactions with supportive oncology, extending beyond access and communication barriers. A relevant example is a Deaf person may prefer for an interpreter in clinic (a reasonable adjustment) and are confident in their Deaf identity to assert their right to privacy in healthcare, rather than using family as interpreters. A deaf person due to cancer or anti-cancer treatment may prefer more support from family during healthcare consultations, as they adjust to a new perspective. See Box 7.1.

BOX 7.1: POINTS FOR CONSIDERATION WHEN CARING FOR D/DEAF PERSONS

d/Deaf Persons Prior to Cancer Diagnosis or Anti-Cancer Treatment	Deaf Persons Due to Cancer or Anti-Cancer Treatment
Recognize that the d/Deaf person is an expert about how a cancer diagnosis may impact on their d/Deaf identity	May need support in adjusting to new experiences and identity as a deaf person with physical, social, and psychological consequences
Ask the d/Deaf person about their preferred communication method during consultations, and for all correspondence	Likely to understand written English fluently, so may prefer written information or videos in spoken English with captions
More likely to obtain healthcare information from within their own d/Deaf community	May need guidance and support with practical adaptations such as hearing aids
Likely to have experienced significant health inequalities already	May be encountering health inequalities related to deafness and cancer for the first time

Supportive oncology teams should employ shared decision-making and individualized patient-centred care protocol to improve care for Deaf patients. Recently, there have been encouraging examples of improving access to authoritative healthcare information in BSL by independent sector organizations such as the Macmillan Deaf Cancer Support Project.[33] The primary message that "Deaf people are the experts on how to communicate with Deaf people" is not only a powerful invitation for collaboration, but also to co-design services to deliver culturally and linguistically appropriate healthcare for Deaf persons.

Under the 2010 Equality Act, the "duty to make reasonable adjustments for disabled people" includes providing written information in accessible formats such as large print or audio format.[7] Persons registered as sight impaired (SS) or severely sight impaired (SSI) report significant challenges with not only accessing healthcare information in suitable formats, but also experiencing inequitable healthcare treatment due to delays in obtaining accessible format information, and worries about requesting appropriate communication support, often resulting in the individual giving up attempting to request the necessary support.[34] Similarly, people with SI or SSI frequently rely on friends or family members to read aloud personal and confidential healthcare information which may cause complications with confidentiality and privacy. They are also often unable to receive basic information such as outpatient appointment details or letters in accessible formats, so there is a very real risk of lack of support and accessible information.

Very little is known about the impact of sight impairment due to cancer or systemic anti-cancer treatment (SACT). Sight impairment due to cancer or cancer treatment can be considered in three broad categories:

1. Primary cancers of the eye or visual tract i.e. ocular melanoma, intra-ocular lymphoma

2. Metastatic cancer and cancer complications i.e. cranial nerve neuropathies due to metastatic infiltrative disease, infections due to immunosuppression

3. Systemic anti-cancer treatment related effects i.e. ocular toxicity from targeted therapies

Although many ocular toxicities due to SACT are low severity, serious complications such as severe or complete sight loss do occur. Whilst physical, social, and psychological complications of sight impairment will vary between individuals, the impact of sight impairment cannot be understated. Supportive oncology teams who encounter patients developing SI or SSI due to cancer and cancer treatment need to offer tailored, individualized care and support to adjust to different ways of living everyday life, as well as potentially accessing healthcare information in new formats such as large print or audio format.

Persons with an intellectual disability represent a diverse and heterogeneous community with different support and communication needs. Persons with an intellectual disability may need support to express physical and psychological symptoms of cancer and cancer treatment, reasonable adjustments to support the delivery of cancer care (such as being accompanied by a family member or carer), and provision of accessible information.

They may communicate in different ways including easy read symbols and text and use communications systems such as Makaton. Providing information in an accessible and understandable format is an essential component of equitable care for persons with an intellectual disability. Research indicates that limited understanding of cancer diagnosis and anti-cancer treatment is a significant concern resulting in high levels of psychological distress.[35] Finally, lack of appropriate information to support the person to understand the signs and symptoms of cancer recurrence compounds the existing inequalities.

Understanding the unique challenges faced by people affected by homelessness and/or disability, and/or who identify as LGBT, and recognizing that these social determinants impact clinical outcomes should be considered good practice in supportive oncology. Whilst this is by no means an exhaustive list of issues that would benefit from an intersectional approach, as the numbers of people living with and beyond cancer increases, the need to tackle health inequalities from a holistic and person-centred perspective has never been greater. Similarly, the need to provide joined up services, from acute to primary health services, social services, and through the voluntary and community-based sector to support clinical teams is critical to delivering good outcomes and improving patient experiences. Finally, these ambitions must be supported by a legislative framework that comprehensively champions human rights, equality, inclusion, and diversity at all levels of society.

References

1. World Health Organization. Promoting health and reducing health inequities by addressing the social determinants of health [internet], 2016; available at: http://www.euro.who.int/__data/assets/pdf_file/0016/141226/Brochure_promoting_health.pdf (accessed Dec 2022).
2. United Nations. Transforming our world: the 2030 agenda for sustainable development [intenet], 2015; available at: https://sustainabledevelopment.un.org/post2015/ transformingourworld (accessed Dec 2022).
3. Department of Health and Social Care, NHS Constitution for England [internet], 2015; available at: https://www.gov.uk/government/publications/the-nhs-constitution-for-england (accessed Dec 2022).
4. NHS. Five Year Forward View [internet], 2014; available at: https://www.england.nhs.uk/wp-content/uploads/2014/10/5yfv-web.pdf (accessed Dec 2022).
5. NHS. The long term plan[internet], 2019; available at: www.longtermplan.nhs.uk (accessed Dec 2022).

6. Heaslip V, Nadaf C. Diversity and Health Inequalities: the role of the practice nurse. *Practice Nursing*. 2019;30:596–599.
7. UK Government. Equality Act 2010: guidance; available at: https://www.gov.uk/guidance/equality-act-2010-guidance (accessed Feb 2023).
8. State Council Information Office, Gender Equality and Women's Development [internet], 2005; available at: http://www.china.org.cn/english/2005/Aug/139404.htm#10.
9. Campinha-Bacote J. Cultural competency: a paradigm shift in the cultural competence versus cultural humility debate – part I. *OJIN* 2018;24(1).
10. Ministry of Human Resources and Social Security. Notice … on further regulating recruitment practices to promote women's employment [internet], 2019; available at: https://www.mohrss.gov.cn/SYrlzyhshbzb/jiuye/zcwj/201902/t20190221_310707.html.
11. Dunn DS, Andrews EE. Person-first and identity-first language: developing psychologists' cultural competence using disability language. *Am Psychol* 2015;70(3):255–264.
12. Crenshaw K. Demarginalizing the intersection of race and sex: a black feminist critique of antidiscrimination doctrine, feminist theory, and antiracist politics. *University of Chicago Leg Forum* 1989;140:139–167.
13. Kapilashrami, A, Hankivsky O. Intersectionality and why it matters to global health. *The Lancet* 2018;391(10140):2589–2591.
14. Holman D et al. Can intersectionality help with understanding and tackling health inequalities? Perspectives of professional stakeholders. *Health Res Policy Syst*. 2021;19:97.
15. UK Government. Homelessness code of guidance for local authorities, 2018; available at: https://www.gov.uk/guidance/homelessness-code-of-guidance-for-local-authorities/chapter-6-homeless-or-threatened-with-homelessness (accessed Mar 2023).
16. Henwood BF et al. Examining mortality among formerly homeless adults enrolled in housing first: an observational study. *BMC Public Health* 2015;15(1):1209.
17. White J et al. Mortality among rough sleepers, squatters, residents of homeless shelters or hotels and sofa-surfers: a pooled analysis of UK birth cohorts. *Int J Epidemiol* 2022;51(3):839–846.
18. Morrison DS. Homelessness as an independent risk factor for mortality: results from a retrospective cohort study. *Int J Epidemiol* 2009;38(3):877–883.
19. Vijayaraghavan M et al. Health, access to health care, and health care use among homeless women with a history of intimate partner violence. *J Community Health* 2012;37(5):1032–1039.
20. Kohler RE et al. Trauma and cervical cancer screening among women experiencing homelessness: a call for trauma-informed care. *Women's Health* 2021;17.
21. Odoh C. et al. Association of fear and mistrust with stress among sheltered homeless adults and the moderating effects of race and sex. *J Racial Ethnic Health Disparities* 2020;7(3):458–467.
22. Garey L et al. Health-related quality of life among homeless smokers: risk and protective factors of latent class membership. *Behav Med* 2019;45(1):40–51.
23. Cimino T et al. Psychosocial distress among oncology patients in the safety net. *PsychoOncology* 2020[29(11):1927–1935.
24. Tobin J. et al. Hospice care access inequalities: a systematic review and narrative synthesis. *BMJ Support Palliat Care* 2022;12(2):142–151.
25. Ivers JH. et al. Five-year standardised mortality ratios in a cohort of homeless people in Dublin. *BMJ Open* 2019;9(1):e023010.
26. Ralph S. Developing UK guidance on how long men should abstain from receiving anal sex before, during and after interventions for prostate cancer. *Clin Oncol*. 2021;33(12):807–810.
27. Griffin L et al. Sex, gender and gender identity: a re-evaluation of the evidence. *Br J Psych Bulletin* 2021;45(5):291–299.
28. Dhejne C et al. Mental health and gender dysphoria: a review of the literature. *Int Rev Psychiatry* 2016;28:44–57.
29. Trans Legislation Tracker; available at: https://translegislation.com/ (accessed Mar 2023).
30. Gender Identity Development Service. Referrals to GIDS. GIRES, 2020; available at https://www.gires.org.uk/tavistock-gender-identity-development-service-data/ (accessed Mar 2023).

31. British Deaf Association, Statistics [internet]; available at: https://bda.org.uk/help-resources/ #statistics (accessed Dec 2022).

32. Macmillan Deaf Cancer Support Project; available at: https://deafcancersupport.org.uk/ (accessed Feb 2023).

33. Royal National Institute for the Blind. Communication Failure? Review of the accessibility of health information for blind and partially sighted people in Scotland [internet], 2020; available at: https://media.rnib.org.uk/documents/Communication_Failure.pdf (accessed Mar 2023).

34. Flynn S et al. "You don't know what's wrong with you": an exploration of cancer-related experiences in people with an intellectual disability. *PsychoOncology* 2016:25;1198–1205.

35. Hung J. Gender equality in China. *OxHRH Blog*, 9 Sept 2017; available at: https://ohrh.law.ox .ac.uk/gender-equality-in-china (accessed Dec 2022).

Section V

Organizational Changes

8

Reviewing Relationships with Palliative and End-of-Life Care

Jennifer Vidrine, Sam H. Ahmedzai, and Richard Berman

Palliative care is an approach that improves the quality of life of patients (adults and children) and their families who are facing problems associated with life-threatening illness. It prevents and relieves suffering through the early identification, correct assessment and treatment of pain and other problems, whether physical, psychosocial or spiritual.

(WHO, 2014[1])

Inception of Palliative Care

In 1967, the late Dame Cicely Saunders founded the first modern hospice, St Christopher's in London. With it came the conception of the modern hospice movement. The aim was to provide a space in which patients with a 'terminal' condition had access to care focused on improving quality of life and symptomatic relief, often felt to be of secondary importance by the treating clinicians of the time.[2] The term 'palliative care' was later coined by Canadian urological surgeon Balfour Mount to give a name to care that did not seek to hasten or prolong death but offered multidisciplinary support for patients with a life-limiting condition, helping them to live well before they died.

The learning and development of practice, particularly around pain and the use of opiates and pioneering in its time, provides much of the basis on which we manage pain in life-limiting conditions today. Initially, there was a focus on patients with a cancer diagnosis[2] and this was invariably in the context of patients in whom any systemic anti-cancer therapies available were not appropriate and in whom death was likely to be imminent. This hospice, and those that subsequently opened around the world, were almost entirely charitably funded. It remains the case that a significant amount of the resources directed at the delivery of palliative and end-of-life care comes from the third sector with only a proportion being funded by central government.

Throughout the next four decades, the speciality of palliative care evolved and expanded, increasingly recognizing the need to address the symptomatic and end-of-life care needs of those with non-malignant disease such as respiratory failure and neurological conditions. There are now established palliative care teams supporting care in hospitals globally. In addition, community palliative care teams often play an integral part in supporting

DOI: 10.1201/9781003369912-17

the care delivered by primary care teams to those with life-limiting and life-threatening conditions.

Today, there exists a large amount of heterogeneity and variation in what is available for patients. One example of this from the UK is access to 24/7 palliative care support as mandated by the Care Quality Commission (CQC) core service framework for end-of-life care.[3] This is only available in 60% of UK trusts and leads to a 'postcode lottery' in which some patients receive a more comprehensive and enveloping service than others, dependent entirely on where they live. The national audit for care at end-of-life (NACEL) 2019/20 reported that two-thirds of hospitals in England and Wales lacked face-to-face comprehensive specialist palliative care leaving patients without the specialist input they need.[4]

A growing evidence base highlights how access to palliative and end-of-life care is significantly impacted by factors including ethnicity, socioeconomic status, and geographic location.[5] The speciality has much to do in ensuring these inequalities are addressed and that equity of care exists for all those in need. In 2022, the UK Government legislated that palliative and end-of-life care should be universally available through the new Integrated Care Boards (Health and Care Act 2022). It remains to be seen how this ideal translates into actual practice. Health inequalities in relation to supportive oncology have been discussed earlier in this book.

Why Modern Oncology Is Challenging Traditional Palliative Care

The cancer landscape has changed almost beyond recognition since the 1960s. Significant advances in cancer therapies, including novel and targeted treatments, have revolutionized patient outcomes and experiences, even in those with metastatic disease which previously would have likely conferred a poor prognosis. Patients with diseases such as metastatic breast, colon, and malignant melanoma have seen their potential life expectancy increase by many years, although the survivorship story is not duplicated across all disease types. As introduced at the beginning of this book, the challenges of living with active but managed disease and/or the consequences of treatment are now increasingly recognized. People with cancer are now living for much longer (even with incurable disease) with a rising number of cancer survivors. Provision of excellent care at the end-of-life remains hugely important, although in comparison to incidence, the number of deaths from cancer in the UK has reported a less dramatic increase. There are new and emerging challenges associated with how we support increasingly complex problems associated with the disease and its treatments. In this new and rapidly changing demographic, could established palliative care services flex and adapt to ensure that the needs of patients with a cancer diagnosis are being met universally across the whole continuum of the disease (including survivorship), rather than exclusively concentrating on care in the end-of-life phase?

Barriers to Change

Any change in mindset and approach to better align existing services with a changing landscape can be fraught with obstacles.

Appropriateness of National Drivers

After the withdrawal of the Liverpool Care Pathway in 2014 it was clear that there needed to be more robust, evidence-based policy and guidance on how to support patients with palliative and end-of-life care needs, particularly those in the last days of life. In 2019, NICE published its guidance "NG142 End of Life Care for Adults: Service Delivery" in which recommendations were made around care standards including the importance of holistic needs assessments.[6] This broadened the scope of the end-of-life phase, referring now to the estimated final 12 months of life, and recognizing the role that advance care planning plays in empowering individuals with the opportunity to plan for their future care. For a patient with cancer, in which it is increasingly clear that earlier intervention can bring major benefits, this mandate to provide holistic, multidisciplinary care at a stage much earlier than just the last days or weeks of life represents a sea-change in practice. Interventions such as Emergency Healthcare Plans and the ReSPeCT initiative reflect a decade of work from the palliative care community to address these changes. Similarly, Advanced Care Planning is now a huge focus in palliative care, although some still question its validity.[7]

The disease trajectory of patients with cancer has changed over the last couple of decades not least due to the significant amount of prognostic uncertainty that novel treatments can bring. A sound understanding of these trajectories, with appreciation of all the nuance involved, is crucial to ensure conversations with patients are safe and effective. Do palliative care professionals possess this understanding and experience to inform the advance care planning they are supporting on these new therapies? (Novel therapies for the management of pain, symptoms, and late consequences of treatment are discussed earlier in this book.)

An additional challenge in prognostication in those with cancer is the recognized treatment-related side effects that some interventions can bring. These can manifest in a clinical change or deterioration that has the risk of being confused by the well-intentioned non-specialist as part of a dying process, as opposed to a potentially reversible situation, caused by the very drugs aiming to prolong a patient's life. In situations such as this, steroids are required (not opioids); however, there can then be a move to initiating symptomatic medications including those that can be sedating, potentially clouding the picture further.

Outcome Measures and Resource Allocation

Demonstrating the impact and value of palliative care brings challenges. Overcoming these is essential in securing resources and support in health systems without limitless supplies of either. The need to show 'benefit' and cost effectiveness has also brought a focus on easily measurable outcomes, particularly cost-saving ones which include the measure of 'preferred and actual place of dying'. This quality measure is increasingly recognized as being less than ideal, not least in patients who go on to die with conditions such as acute leukaemia in whom a death in hospital, even in the critical care environment, would be felt to be unavoidable. It is also entirely possible to support goal-concordant care that includes a death in hospital. The need to shift focus from 'place of care' to 'quality of care' is increasingly acknowledged, with an awareness that one does not ensure the other.[8]

A growing body of work on patient-reported outcome measures (PROMs) recognizes the need to ensure that it is the patient and those close to them who discern the efficacy of our services, not the healthcare professionals delivering them. Initiatives such as the Outcome

Assessment and Complexity Collaborative (OACC) suite of measures in which patients are invited to participate in answering validated questionnaires about their needs and experiences are now in use by an increasing number of palliative care services around the country.[9] Further research into which outcome measures are the most appropriate, useful, and patient centred is imperative if palliative care teams are going to effectively contribute to the delivery of a well-funded, holistic supportive care service for patients with a cancer diagnosis. We must not continue in burdening patients with the same measures we have used for years, without pausing to consider their drawbacks and to critically weigh up their relevance in the modern cancer world.

Resource restraints are often cited as one of the major concerns about any evolution of the traditional palliative care model to better meet the needs of patients with cancer. There is a widely held anxiety that palliative care teams broadening their remit and scope will 'open the floodgates' of referrals to such an extent that will be unmanageable. Being able to demonstrate to policy makers and NHS leaders the inherent benefit and economic sense of a supportive care approach opens important opportunities for potential cost savings.

Traditionally Effective Models of Palliative Care

Since its inception in the 1960s, palliative care has generally focused on those patients for whom curative treatment is no longer an option and instead a new phase of 'palliative' interventions has commenced. This traditional, dichotomous view in which patients are seen as in either a 'curable' or 'palliative' group has become increasingly obsolete for many.

Patients are experiencing growing amounts of uncertainty inherent in undergoing novel treatments and often even their treating teams are not entirely sure what the response to these may be, nor even if a long-term remission or 'cure' may be possible.

On the other hand, as discussed above, even those patients with advancing and metastatic disease, who a few decades ago were regarded as 'dying', can now live for many more years, and with this in mind, and the availability and appropriateness of local resources and/or referral pathways, clinicians can struggle with the appropriate timing of a referral to palliative care.

Emerging evidence highlights the clear role for earlier, upstream, and more proactive palliation-directed care, especially in groups such as those with haematological malignancies, who are heavily symptomatic but in which these uncertainties are even more pronounced. In addition, those undergoing intensive therapies such as stem cell transplants have been shown to have reduced psychological morbidity and improved quality of life when offered routine and embedded access to palliative care teams,[10–12] even though these high-stake interventions are risky and undertaken with curative intent.

Patients and those close to them are living with 'treatable but incurable' cancers in which a 'palliative' label has, due to the incurable nature of their condition, been comfortably applied. They often have reason to expect significantly longer prognoses than previously had been the case, often over several years. They are, however, often living with the burden of many symptomatic, psychological, and social challenges.

There are real problems with drawing from a model in which tried and tested palliative care interventions are used liberally. Some of the dangers include the overuse of long-term use of medications such as opioids, arguably the 'go to' drug class of choice for palliative care clinicians, and applying traditional palliative care approaches to patients who are considered "living with and beyond cancer".

Do palliative care teams have the necessary training and experience and is there the research and evidence available to underpin alternative methods of managing symptoms?

In many cancer centres, services have evolved in such a way that it is often palliative care-trained physicians and teams that are positioned and expected to provide the holistic supportive care to patients with cancer. Some individuals have taken opportunities to critically appraise what is on offer and whether it is meeting the right needs at the right time working collaboratively with other services. Others may be more wedded to a more traditional model, showing reluctance to upskill, flex, or adapt to what patients tell us they need and therefore be more reluctant/unwilling to be involved in the care of those without a clear 'palliative' prognosis.

Training and Education

It has generally been assumed that those with palliative care credentials and training are most appropriately set up to co-ordinate the delivery of the supportive care described throughout this textbook. Core skillsets such as the ability to undertake skilled bio/psycho/social assessment and have sensitive conversations about the direction of future care bring much to the table. However, the opportunities that exist within palliative care training at both undergraduate and postgraduate level are scarce and many of those acquiring a certificate in completion of training (CCT) in palliative care and then go on to work in a palliative care service have had very little access to any formal training on the newly emerging needs as described above. Until recently, there was no national network of shared practice and support and little consensus on how to manage commonly encountered symptoms, such as oral mucositis secondary to treatments.

Similarly, in the primary care setting, GPs leading on the delivery of holistic care for those with cancer are even less likely to have had training in supportive oncology. Modern supportive oncology requires a new skillset and a different approach with input from the full range of supporting medical and non-medical specialties. The problems faced even by those with metastatic disease can last for many years and it does not seem appropriate or feasible that oncologists or palliative care physicians alone will continue to remain the sole providers of care for those with supportive oncology needs in the long term.

Research, Guidelines, and Protocols

Presently, there is a dearth of research or evidence-based guidance of how to manage the extensive and rapidly broadening range of supportive and palliative care needs of people affected by cancer. Although palliative care has, for some years, benefited from conferences, networking, reference guides, and textbooks, these have traditionally not included specific information on the management of patients with treatment toxicities and uncertain or longer prognoses. Perhaps there has even been an element of 'making it up as we go along'. The inception of the UK Association for Supportive Care in Cancer (UKASCC) in the early 2020s was a milestone in establishing a community of practice, dovetailing with several existing organizations around the world including the Multinational Association of Supportive Care in Cancer (MASCC). A stated aim of UKASCC is to try and address the lack of research happening in the arena of supportive care by supporting teams to actively seek out opportunities to engage in research in the field.

End-of-Life Care

This chapter is a manifesto that patients with a cancer diagnosis have a right to and can benefit from proactive and early-intervention supportive care with involvement from suitably trained palliative care teams. There exists a societal understanding of the association of palliative care with death and dying, and yet, as outlined earlier in this chapter, many of the patients seen by modern palliative care teams are not imminently dying. However, it is also true that many of the patients with a cancer diagnosis will go on to die of their cancer. Therefore, a supportive care service offering 'whole pathway' support from the point of diagnosis until whatever comes next must be willing and able to support end-of-life care.

The way in which teams are supported, equipped, and mandated to deliver end-of-life care in both the community and hospital environment has changed significantly, notwithstanding miscalculations such as the roll-out of the Liverpool Care Pathway. In the UK, national documents, such as "one chance to get it right" created by the National Leadership Alliance for the Care of the Dying Person, have shaped how healthcare providers and commissioners have directed funding and resources. Similarly, the Care Quality Commission (CQC) looks specifically at the delivery of end-of-life care within its inspection framework, providing additional impetus for providers to ensure that this care meets expectations.

We now aim to look at how to improve the quality and experience of the life of a person affected by cancer, bolstered by the growing recognition that this needs a broader approach that is beyond just the last phase of someone's life. Whilst palliative care must not lose sight of where it has come from, it must grow, change, and adapt to maintain true 'person-centred' care, whilst also continuing to be alongside patients and their loved ones as they approach the end of their life.

References

1. WHO. Palliative care [internet], 2014; available at: https://www.who.int/news-room/fact-sheets/detail/palliative-care (accessed Oct 2024).
2. Saunders C. The evolution of palliative care. *J Royal Soc Med.* 2001;94(9):430–432.
3. Care Quality Commission. Core service: end of life care [internet]; available at: https://www.cqc.org.uk/sites/default/files/20170629-IH-end-of-life-care-core-service-framework.pdf.
4. National Audit of Care at the End of Life (NACEL) [internet], 2019; available at: https://www.hqip.org.uk/resource/national-audit-of-care-at-the-end-of-life-nacel-2019/ (accessed Sept 2024).
5. UK Government. Palliative and end of life care. *POSTnote* [internet] 2022;675; available at: https://researchbriefings.files.parliament.uk/documents/POST-PN-0675/POST-PN-0675.pdf (accessed Sept 2024).
6. NICE, End of life care for adults: service delivery [internet], 2019; available at: https://www.nice.org.uk/guidance/NG142 (accessed Sept 2024).
7. Jimenez G et al. Overview of systematic reviews of advance care planning: summary of evidence and global lessons. *J Pain Symptom Manage.* 2018;56(3):436–459.e25.
8. Hoare S et al. End-of-life care quality measures: beyond place of death. *BMJ Support Palliat Care.* 2022;3841.
9. Palliative care Outcome Scale (POS) Frequently Asked Questions [internet], 2015; available at https://pos-pal.org/maix/faq.php.

10. El-Jawahri A et al. Effect of inpatient palliative care on quality of life 2 weeks after hematopoietic stem cell transplantation: a randomized clinical trial. *JAMA*. 2016;316(20):2094–2103.
11. El-Jawahri A et al. Effectiveness of integrated palliative and oncology care for patients with acute myeloid leukemia: a randomized clinical trial. *JAMA Oncol*. 2021;7(2):238–245.
12. Rodin G et al. Emotion and symptom-focused engagement (EASE): a randomized phase II trial of an integrated psychological and palliative care intervention for patients with acute leukemia. *Support Care Cancer*. 2020;28(1):163–176.

9

The Future – How Do Services Models Need to Adapt?

Jo Thompson, Emma Dillsworth, Freya Howle, and Oli Minton

Introduction

Delivery of large-scale change in clinical practice has a better chance of being sustained if supported and delivered as a project or programme that is linked to the wider aims of health services in that country.

When trying to get strategic-level endorsement and engagement in transformation, especially within established clinical services such as cancer care, a clear business case must demonstrate how patients will benefit in the short, medium, and long term, and how the project will deliver good value for money.

In the UK, the current climate is prioritizing resources and funding to help recovery of elective (planned care) services by addressing significant backlogs that were seriously exacerbated by the COVID pandemic. A great effort is also being made to increase patient access to new models of care, new treatment options, and holistic, personalized care plans, recognizing that all patients must be supported appropriately both clinically and non-clinically.

Giving a Clear Definition: What Is Supportive Oncology?

Supportive oncology currently describes the co-ordinated contributions of a collective group of medical and non-medical specialties that collectively help to prevent and manage the adverse effects of cancer and its treatments. Supportive oncology spans the entire spectrum of the disease. It includes prehabilitation, management of treatable but incurable cancer, curative disease, survivorship, and palliative and end of life care. The optimal delivery of supportive oncology requires input from a multitude of trained practitioners working in diverse specialties (medical and non-medical, including components of palliative care) to assist accurate diagnosis, comprehensive assessment, holistic management, and ultimately to improve patient outcomes and experience.

DOI: 10.1201/9781003369912-18

There is a growing body of evidence that timely access to supportive treatments can lead to improvements in quality of life and survival, as well as benefitting the health economy. The development of a broad multi-professional basis for the study and expansion of supportive care through the Multinational Association of Supportive Care in Cancer (MASCC) – and more recently through the UK Association of Supportive Care in Cancer (UKASCC) – has been an important step in fostering the growth of an evidence base. MASCC's success has undoubtedly been underpinned by the successful integration of oncological and non-oncological specialties.

Why Now?

Managing cancer and cancer treatment-related morbidity is fast becoming a significant public health and economic challenge. Currently in England, around 1.8 million people are living with a diagnosis of cancer and this number is increasing by over 3% a year. The total figure is set rise to over 3 million by 2030, and 5.2 million by 2040.

Despite the significant progress in oncological treatment, a large proportion of patients who are 'living with cancer' still experience morbidity and symptoms, resulting from the cancer and/or its treatment. Increases in cancer incidence, emergency care hospitalizations, earlier intensive care unit admissions, and treatment costs have all added to the global burden of cancer care. The disease is becoming a major economic expenditure for all developed countries. In the UK and in the USA, cancer care costs are substantial and expected to rise significantly in the future due to growth and aging of the population and improvements in survival, as well as trends in treatment patterns and costs of care following cancer diagnosis.

The availability of supportive care services is inequitable. Currently, many cancer centres in the UK have some level of supportive care services, either because of NHS England's Enhanced Supportive Care (ESC) programme or local initiatives. However, the format of these teams is variable, as are the patient cohort (i.e., restricted to specific cancer diagnoses) and the interventions offered (i.e., often restricted to symptom control).

Strategies for System Developments

The NHS Long Term Plan aims to save thousands more lives each year by dramatically improving how we diagnose and treat cancer. The ambition is that by '2028, an extra 55,000 people each year will survive for five years or more following their cancer diagnosis'.[1]

The 2023/24 cancer priorities and operational planning guidance reconfirm the ongoing need to recover core services and improve productivity as it is recognized that 'prevention and the effective management of long-term conditions are key to improving population health and curbing the ever-increasing demand for healthcare services'.[2]

Integrated Care Boards (ICBs) were legally formed nationwide in July 2022 and whilst the operational governance structures are being continually developed, Cancer Alliances are still formally recognized within them as the cancer delivery arm, who will 'continue to lead whole-system planning and delivery of cancer care ... as well as providing clinical leadership and advice on commissioning'.[3]

Helping to drive forward any strategies for systems to develop innovative approaches to delivering supportive oncology are the planning requirements of ICBs and Cancer Alliances who must submit returns to the national programme.

Working with a "Cancer Alliance" – An Example in Greater Manchester, UK

With the overarching aims of the NHS Long Term Plan and recently published cancer priorities requiring 'holistic needs assessments, a care plan, and health and wellbeing information and support',[1] the emphasis is now on changing attitudes and approaches towards the implementation of these ambitions. The intention is for patients to have more choice and control over the way their care is planned and delivered, based on 'what matters' to them. To achieve this in Greater Manchester, the Cancer Alliance has established a typical "Personalised Care" Programme.

It is hoped the outputs from this programme will inform and provide ICB-level oversight and co-ordination of services, helping to identify what is already being offered to patients, how and where, the quality and usefulness of current services, and most importantly, the gaps in services to be addressed.

This information will inform the development of new referral pathways (or improve access to existing pathways) which can be utilized by supportive oncology MDTs to improve the personalization of their service.

Through targeted funding and co-ordination of service provision, this programme will also reduce the likelihood of duplication of effort across the region, improving the overall return on investment, and offering substantial efficiency savings. It will further the integration of voluntary and community-based services into health systems, and improve communication between primary care and acute settings, helping to reduce health inequalities and promoting cohesion and resilience in local communities.

Undoubtably these are ambitious strategic goals. Health systems in England remain challenged with workforce and financial pressures, long waiting lists, and an aging population likely to put even more pressure on services. It remains to be seen if these advantages can be completely realized.

Developing a Model for Supportive Oncology

Service development needs to be informed by understanding the current offer across the different healthcare sectors including acute and tertiary trusts, commissioned services in primary care, community healthcare offers, voluntary and community sector enterprises, and beyond. Robust demand and capacity modelling will be crucial to remap services to allocate resources with maximum effectiveness.

The benefits of this approach include:

- Informed development of processes across individuals' journeys to establish maximum efficiency and best use of resources
- Effective resource planning to allow more focused delivery of care where it is most needed across a pathway
- Better understanding of the financial impact of demand to make sure services are delivered to their full capacity without exceeding the budget
- More efficient planning for the projected cultural changes in the population and the services individuals will require

What Underpins Successful Transformation?

Developing a new service model and strategy in healthcare will require large-scale culture change which can be supported by crosscutting workstreams including:

- Communication and engagement – the healthcare system and patients will need to know what the service is, its benefits, and how to access it.
- Workforce planning – to ensure that the service is deliverable for patients.
- Education and training – giving healthcare professionals the confidence and skills to deliver the service.

Supportive Oncology: What Does It Look Like in Practice?

There is growing recognition internationally of the need for the integration of supportive oncology into standard oncology services.[4,5] Whilst this recognition and endorsement helps support the case to develop these services, there is currently no 'blueprint' for how they should be operationalized. There are different potential models for supportive care and each new service needs to consider their unique set up, as no single model will be appropriate for all settings.

Most supportive oncology services use an outpatient model made up of a core team of professionals usually (although not exclusively) from within specialist palliative care or oncology teams.[6]

These professionals need to have training in the broad range of skills needed to provide day-to-day care across the whole spectrum of the disease, with critical elements from the main associated allied non-oncology specialties.[7] The clinical care must aim to:

- Provide personalized and targeted treatments consistent with stage of disease
- Focus on preservation and improvement in quality of life
- Affect survival and the quality of that survival
- Permit the use of the most effective anti-cancer agents
- Assist accurate diagnosis and management

Core professionals will generally be consultants and clinical nurse specialists (CNSs) who will carry out initial assessments, plan care, and refer to wider oncology specific services such as dietitians, psychology, and allied health professionals.

For some teams these wider roles may in fact form part of the core. Optimal supportive oncology also requires access to a range of specialties (e.g., endocrinology, rheumatology, acute oncology, dermatology) who work in an integrated and collaborative way, so that patients have access to the range of expertise in managing cancer and cancer treatment-related problems across the whole cancer pathway.

Different models of supportive oncology clinics include the following.

Embedded Clinics

This involves members of the supportive oncology team being present in other site-specific oncology clinics. This has benefits as teams are working from a shared space, which supports integration. Patients will experience teams working together so care may feel less fragmented; they can also see different professionals during one appointment, which can reduce the burden of outpatient visits.

The challenge of this model is that the supportive oncology team would need to be present in multiple site-specific oncology clinics which may present workforce capacity issues. In addition, there may be constraints around available clinic rooms and time within the oncology clinics for supportive oncology teams to review patients. This could in turn limit growth of the service.

Supportive Oncology Clinics

These are stand-alone clinics operating within the cancer centre. Patients receive scheduled appointments with the supportive oncology team either in person or virtually. This model has the advantage of being able to offer support to multiple tumour groups at any stage in the cancer continuum giving patients dedicated time and tailored follow-up within a specific clinic.

Supportive oncology clinics may be consultant-led or nurse-led (some centres also have clinic-based supportive oncology physiotherapy, dietetics, and pharmacy) with the option to access further consultant advice/review if indicated. This is the ideal model as it allows growth and development of services but may be challenging if there is not enough physical space in oncology outpatient departments to support the required activity.

Virtual vs Face-to-Face Consultations

Since the COVID-19 pandemic there has been an increase in telehealth i.e., virtual consultations either by telephone or video. Virtual appointments have the obvious advantage that patients do not need to travel to hospitals or clinics to engage with healthcare professionals. This reduces the financial burden of travel including parking costs as well as time spent in waiting areas of busy clinics. Telehealth also reduces the physical space needed to run clinics.

The disadvantages of telehealth lie in the lack of opportunity for recognizing non-verbal cues from patients and in that it does not enable a physical examination. Perhaps a supportive oncology clinic with options for both virtual and face-to-face appointments represents the best approach.

The Supportive Oncology MDT

The Christie NHS Foundation Trust in Greater Manchester, England, hold bi-weekly meetings where complex cases from across the whole continuum of cancer are discussed and plans are made for ongoing treatment. This meeting comprises the core supportive oncology service, with relevant input from allied specialties (such as endocrinology, surgical, psycho-oncology, rehabilitation, oncology, etc.) who are invited according to the requirements of the case/clinical needs.

Cultural and Institutional Challenges

It appears that most supportive oncology teams come across initial reticence during their early months of practicing. There is sometimes hesitancy from oncologists and site-specific nurse specialists to refer their patients to these services. Why might this be?

Perhaps there is a lack of clarity around what a supportive oncology service can offer that is different to existing services and targeted nursing support. There also could be some confusion about how a supportive oncology service may differ from already well-established palliative care services, particularly if these services have been rebranded as enhanced supportive care.[8] Alternatively, there may be cultural issues within the workforce that create resistance to innovation or accepting changes to established practice.

Alongside highlighting the benefits and principles of supportive oncology to potential sceptics, practical solutions to help with integration have included running embedded clinics (as described above). This is likely to create an atmosphere of trust conducive to encouraging referrals.

A simple and clear referral system that is easy to use is vital. An optimal model could include the use of standardized need-based criteria to trigger a referral for patients who are most appropriate for specialist palliative care in the outpatient setting, allowing for a more personalized approach.[9] Individual services would need to decide if their "triggers" for referral are, for example, symptom based or pre-defined and time based, e.g., all newly diagnosed with locally advanced or metastatic disease. This would also depend on the clinic capacity of the workforce available.

Ease of referral is important. Clinicians can find locating and completing the correct referral forms and information for different services time consuming and inefficient. It can be helpful to just have one point of referral that clinicians can use – a "single point of access" – whether this is simply a dedicated supportive oncology phone number or referral email address.

Sometimes when patients are referred to supportive oncology, it can be at a point when their diagnosis is very new to them, and they are completely overwhelmed with information. Patients are trying to digest not only their diagnosis and what this means for themselves and their families, but they are also having to navigate the different teams and contacts within the oncology system they are now part of. There are often perceived blurred lines between supportive care and acute oncology and patients without the correct information struggle to understand the difference.

Perhaps if patients and their relatives were involved in the early stages of creating a service some of these issues could be mitigated. It is also vital to collect, analyse, and act upon any patient feedback in a timely way. A patient satisfaction questionnaire for instance can be an easy way of collecting qualitative data and reviewing the service.

Patients and relatives can find knowing which team to contact for different issues or problems difficult. This points to the fact that patients need clear and specific information from the beginning of their diagnosis detailing what each team does and who to contact. This could be in the form of straightforward patient information leaflets containing relevant contact numbers or access to relevant patient information videos about the team and what they do. Alongside paper copies of information, a bespoke supportive oncology app for use on a smart device such as a mobile phone or tablet may be beneficial to some patients and provide an easy way of accessing information and sign posting to resources specifically tailored for their needs.[10]

One of the areas that supportive oncology can excel at is tailoring the level of input a patient requires during their time with the service. Due to the early referral of patients in their cancer continuum and the fact that most are still having anti-cancer treatment, patients often need different levels of support at different times.

Most patients will want to be an active participant in decisions around their care over a longer period and be involved in how often they are required to be seen. Shared decision making describes the involvement of patients and clinicians working together through sharing of information and reaching a joint consensus for care decisions.[11]

One solution as highlighted in Chapter 4A is to use a Patient-Initiated Follow-Up (PIFU) system whereby patients refer themselves back into the service as new issues arise without the need for a re-referral from another clinician. Running regular clinics throughout the week can also be beneficial to patients who appreciate the ability to be flexible around their other appointments.

Workforce Education, Training, and Retention

One of the biggest challenges facing the design and ongoing operational integrity of clinical services around the world is around identifying, educating, and retaining an effective workforce. Supportive oncology is an evolving area of practice, so skilled clinicians are drawn largely from palliative care and medical/clinical oncology.

In the UK, supportive oncology services are structured differently and have a variety of core members, and this variation in service delivery models has been cited as one of the limitations of enhanced supportive care. It has also been identified that a successful supportive oncology team needs access to the expertise of a wider MDT alongside a dedicated core team.[12] This leads to the question of what should a supportive oncology team look like – who should the key professionals be? Looking at a more long-term vision, a dedicated "core team" would ideally be available in each setting, providing supportive oncology on a day-to-day basis, covering the whole cancer spectrum. The core team would be specialists in the field and would require specific and ongoing supportive oncology education and training. Ultimately, the goal would be for the core team to work collaboratively with and refer to other specialist teams both within and outside of oncology. Examples could include endocrinology or diabetes teams.

One example is the University Hospitals Plymouth NHS Trust "Enhanced Supportive Care" service which employs Allied Health Professionals providing core MDT expertise:

specialist dietitians, counsellors, physiotherapists, and occupational therapists all have a key role to play, alongside medics and nurses.

Undoubtably, these specialisms can offer important perspectives for patients who are being seen in clinic from the point of diagnosis onwards. Where patients are receiving SACT or other anti-cancer treatments, consideration should be given to incorporating input from medical and clinical oncologists. Equally, staff working in supportive oncology should be encouraged to access relevant continuing professional development (CPD) programmes, aimed at supporting gaps in their knowledge and experience.

In the longer term, how might knowledge, training, and professional development be accessed more widely? As the specialty of supportive oncology matures, one might conceivably design virtual knowledge "hubs", where clinicians can access information on a range of topics and where best practice guidelines could be developed. Associations like MASCC, UKASCC, or the NHS Futures Platform are ideally placed to facilitate this.

Patient-Reported Outcome Measures (PROMs)

PROMs allow clinicians to measure and track patients' quality of life, to identify and focus on the issues and outcomes that matter to individuals, as well as to prioritize limited clinical capacity according to the needs of all patients. Remote collection of PROMs aids in triaging and prioritizing patients for clinical review, and results in focused consultations and increased patient satisfaction.[13]

The integration of PROMs into routine clinical care has been shown to increase survival for patients, through a combination of early recognition and targeted intervention, or adjustments to treatment allowing patients to tolerate systemic anti-cancer therapy for longer.[14]

Reviewing PROMs prior to clinic appointments could help tailor interactions and aid clinicians in supportive oncology clinics – e.g., enquiring about psychological wellbeing, which is often overlooked in a busy clinic appointment.[14] Recording PROMs focuses patients on their own symptom burden and can provide a visual representation of this trend over time. This increases information available to clinicians to aid in shared decision making – a priority with recently updated guidelines.[15]

In the UK, feasibility studies had already shown that electronic PROMs are acceptable to most patients locally at the Sussex Cancer Centre, including those who are less digitally engaged.[16]

In September 2020, University Hospitals Sussex NHS Foundation Trust (UHS) implemented a trial, where patients with cancer who could benefit from earlier access to supportive oncology were identified by staff on acute wards. These patients were offered the use of the My Clinical Outcomes (MCO) web-app.

MCO is a patient- and clinician-facing web-platform for remote, long-term collection and real-time analysis of PROMs.

As part of this trial, MCO was configured to prompt patients by email to complete three PROMs assessments routinely every 2 weeks (but they could do so more frequently if desired). Results and progress were made available in real-time to the clinical team and were available for patients themselves to track. The PROMs included were:

- EORTC QLQ-C30 – a 30-question assessment of health-related quality of life for people living with cancer focusing on common physical, financial, social, cognitive, and emotional impacts of disease.[17]
- EQ-5D-3L and EQ-5D VAS – a 5-question assessment of mobility, self-care, ability to continue usual activities, pain/discomfort, and anxiety/depression – a visual analogue scale.[18]

In this study, patients benefitted from 5% fewer unplanned admissions with hospital stays also shorter by an average of 1.43 days. Furthermore, the results showed a return on investment with a benefit cost ratio of 1.4. This is important for commissioners to be able to continue to fund services knowing the system gains overall from any investment. A further analysis suggested that if the service were expanded for the South-East region the programme would deliver approximate savings of £11.2m over the course of 5 years.[19]

At the time of writing work is underway to integrate MCO with University Hospitals Sussex and Sussex ICS systems with a plan to expand the scope and make the technology available to help support more patients in the region.

Supportive Oncology Service in Practice: A Case Study

Jackie, a 69-year-old woman, previously fit and well, was diagnosed with inoperable cholangiocarcinoma. She and her family (husband and two sons) were devastated at her diagnosis and prognosis which was estimated to be around 12 months. She was referred to the enhanced supportive care (ESC) team just prior to starting chemotherapy.

Her first appointment was a face-to-face appointment with a CNS introducing the service and explaining the support available. She had no problematic symptoms but was anxious about the future. Jackie received 8 cycles of chemotherapy and then a period of surveillance; at 12 months her disease was stable. A further scan at 15 months showed progressive disease in the liver.

Throughout this period, she received scheduled monthly phone calls from the ESC nurse. This level of care was implemented (rather than PIFU) considering her prognosis and knowledge of the disease trajectory which would most likely require dedicated input from the ESC team.

She used a dedicated ESC app to send PROMs before her appointments allowing her nurse to monitor if specific issues were bothering her and would warrant more detailed discussion. She also contacted the team on two occasions 'ad hoc' with questions about her symptoms and was able to speak with her nurse.

In addition, Jackie was linked in with the ESC occupational therapist for support with fatigue management. Jackie described the ESC team as her 'safety net' and felt well supported knowing she had scheduled calls. Shortly after the identification of progressive disease, Jackie reported increasing symptoms of abdominal pain, bloating, and constipation at her telephone appointment.

It was agreed that a face-to-face review was warranted. She was booked into the consultant ESC clinic a few days later, from where she was admitted due to evidence of ascites and uncontrolled pain. The ESC team were then able to liaise with her oncology team, review her as an inpatient, manage her symptoms, and talk to her about her future preferences and priorities including where she wanted to be cared for which was, if possible, at home. Unfortunately, Jackie's condition deteriorated throughout this admission. The ESC team liaised with community services and with the support of the ward staff she was transferred home to die with her family.

Through being referred to the ESC team at diagnosis and receiving routine follow-up Jackie was supported by the team throughout her whole cancer journey including at the end of life. The ability to arrange a prompt face-to-face appointment in the ESC clinic following a change in symptoms meant she avoided admission via the emergency department and benefitted from continuity of care from one clinical team.

Artificial Intelligence (AI)

As healthcare data becomes increasingly digitized and familiarity with advances in deep learning technology increases, the opportunities for AI to improve the diagnosis and treatment for cancer become clearer.

An AI tool that can predict the likelihood of a patient encountering late bowel toxicities based on a set of personalized risk factors (as discussed in Chapter 4B) could rapidly improve the clinical risk stratification of patients whilst ensuring, with some certainty, that appropriate mitigations are in place to minimize the impact of future adverse outcomes throughout treatment.

The practical application of AI across healthcare is in its infancy. Developers will undoubtably tailor their products to be simple and easy to use but compatibility with existing systems may be a complicating factor. Will uncertainty amongst healthcare professionals around the effectiveness of the technology stifle innovation? It seems likely that despite a growing number of clinical champions, there will be an influential cohort of sceptics. Is there a chance that AI used as a diagnostic tool would result in a greater incidence of over- or under-diagnosis? What will patients think about the new technology? Will patients and professional attitudes change as their exposure to AI increases?[20] As early as September 2021, there had been at least 64 AI-based medical devices and algorithms approved by the US Food and Drug Administration[21] and despite the high initial costs of implementation, the economic case for greater AI-driven automation across healthcare is undeniable. It seems certain that cancer services will become part of the forthcoming AI-revolution.

Conclusion

Put simply, supportive oncology services help patients to live as well as possible throughout their cancer treatment and beyond. There is growing recognition internationally for the ongoing development of these services; however, the challenge comes from a lack of evidence or guidance as to the most effective delivery model, and how best to integrate new and potentially disruptive technology such as AI.

Most services will include a core of professionals (generally consultants and clinical nurse specialists) who will have access to other specialties within and outside of oncology. Key considerations when developing these services include strategies for communication and engagement with the wider oncology team (this will involve clear explanation as to the purpose and benefits of supportive oncology), workforce, education, and training. Clear and straightforward referral pathways are vital for other teams to engage. Environmental aspects such as physical clinic space within the cancer centre will often dictate which model is best suited to a particular service.

The increasing use of dedicated technology has provided more options for services to fit the needs of patients, for example, virtual consultations, collection of PROMs, dedicated apps, and educational videos. Developing services with input from patients in the form of carefully formulated patient feedback questionnaires will better enable supportive oncology teams to reflect the needs of the population they aim to support.

References

1. NHS. The long-term plan [internet], 2019; available at: www.longtermplan.nhs.uk (accessed Dec 2022).
2. NHS. 2023/24 priorities and operational planning guidance [internet], 2023; available at: https://www.england.nhs.uk/wp-content/uploads/2022/12/PRN00021-23-24-priorities-and -operational-planning-guidance-v1.1.pdf (accessed Aug 2023).
3. NHS. Working together at scale: guidance on provider collaboratives [internet], 2021; available at: https://www.england.nhs.uk/wp-content/uploads/2021/06/B0754-working-together -at-scale-guidance-on-provider-collaboratives.pdf (accessed Aug 2023).
4. Berman R et al. The rise of supportive oncology: a revolution in cancer care. *Clin Oncol.* 2023;35(4):213–215.
5. Hui D et al. Models of supportive care in oncology. *Curr Opin Oncol.* 2021;33(4):259–266.
6. Monnery D et al. Delivery models and health economics of supportive care services in England: A multicentre analysis. *Clin Oncol.* 2023;35(6):e395–e403.
7. Berman R, Davies A. Supportive care is broader than palliative care [corrected]. *Br Med J.* 2019;365:l629.
8. Hui D et al. Improving patient and caregiver outcomes in oncology: team-based, timely, and targeted palliative care. *CA Cancer J Clin.* 2018;68(5):356–376.
9. Health Innovation Kent Surrey Sussex, Bridging the Gap [internet], 2023; available at: https:// healthinnovation-kss.com/bridging-the-gap/new-app-designed-to-better-support-people -living-with-metastatic-cancer-a-case-study/ (accessed May 2023).
10. Bennett R et al. Exploration of shared decision making in oncology within the United States: a scoping review. *Supportive Care Cancer.* 2022;31(1):94.
11. Berman R et al. Supportive care: an indispensable component of modern oncology. *Clin Oncol.* 2020;32(11):781–788.
12. Marandino L et al. COVID-19 emergency and the need to speed up the adoption of electronic patient-reported outcomes in cancer clinical practice. *JCO Oncology Practice.* 2020;16(6):295–298.
13. Basch E et al. Overall survival results of a trial assessing patient-reported outcomes for symptom monitoring during routine cancer treatment. *JAMA.* 2017;318(2):197–198.
14. Crockett C, et al. The routine clinical implementation of electronic patient-reported outcome measures (ePROMs) at the Christie NHS foundation trust. *Clin Oncol.* 2021; 33(12):761–764.
15. NICE. Shared decision making, guideline 197 [internet], 2021; available at: https://www. nice.org.uk/guidance/ng197/resources/shared-decision-making-pdf-66142087186885 (accessed Aug 2023).
16. Appleyard SE et al. Digital medicine in men with advanced prostate cancer – a feasibility study of electronic patient-reported outcomes in patients on systemic treatment. *Clin Oncol.* 2021;33(12):751–760.

17. Aaronson NK et al. The European organisation for research and treatment of cancer QLQ-C30: a quality-of-life instrument for use in international clinical trials in oncology. *JNCI.* 1993;85:365–376.

18. Rabin R, de Charro F. EQ-5D: a measure of health status from the EuroQol group. *Ann Med.* 2001;33(5):337–43.

19. Stewart E et al. Cancer centre supportive oncology service: health economic evaluation. *BMJ Support Palliat Care.* 2022;3716.

20. Benjamens S et al. The state of artificial intelligence-based FDA-approved medical devices and algorithms: an online database. *NPJ Digit Med.* 2020;3:118.

21. Young AT et al. Patient and general public attitudes towards clinical artificial intelligence: a mixed methods systematic review. *The Lancet.* 2021;3(9):599–611.

Index